M000248205

LIVING PROOF

Judith A. Conte with Marianne Del Guercio

MIGHTY
ACORN
PRESS

Living Proof ©2021 by Judith A. Conte.

All rights reserved. No part of this book may be used, reproduced, distributed, or transmitted in any form or by any means whatsoever without the prior written permission of the publisher except for brief quotations in the context of critical reviews and certain other noncommercial uses permitted by copyright law.

livingproofstory.com
ISBN: 978-0-578-58016-6
Printed in USA

Mighty Acorn Press
Anchorage • Chicago

DEDICATED TO JOHN DEL GUERCIO

AUTHOR'S NOTE

This book is the result of a deep dive I took into the lives of my cousin, Marianne Del Guercio, her husband, Rick, and their children, Amber, Britney, Robby, and John. The story you are about to read is true based on individual and collective memories with dialogue that is representative and as best remembered. Characters are real not composite; a few use their actual names. Information presented about Spinal Muscular Atrophy is not intended as medical advice and ought to not be taken as such.

CONTENTS

LIVING PROOF

AUGUST 8, 2002

ANTICIPATION

The twins, identical to everyone except themselves, gather up cereal, milk, bowls, and spoons.

"I'm so glad Mom's having the baby today," Amber says.

"Shush." Britney nudges her sister. "She's coming." Marianne shuffles in followed by the family's two dogs.

"You talkin' about me?" The girls roll their eyes. "I saw that." She kisses each of them in turn. "Are you ready to meet your new baby brother?"

"Yeah," they say in unison.

"Whose name is ...." Marianne drum rolls her fingers on the countertop. "... John Donato Del Guercio."

"Donato?" Amber says.

"That was my Uncle Danny's name. He helped raise me after my father died."

Vera stands at the doorway with her grandson. "Aren't you supposed to be at the hospital?"

Marianne reaches down to hug Robby. "How's my handsome boy this morning?"

"Don't you have an appointment?"

"Yes, you know we do, but we're running late."

Vera gives her daughter a wry smile. "You mean you're running late. I'm sure that husband of yours is waiting for you."

"I love how you always stick up for Rick," Marianne whines, pretending to be upset.

"You better get going unless you want the baby born here."

"All right, all right." She kisses her mother's cheek. "Thanks for watching the kids. With any luck, I'll be back in three days." She almost chokes on the words.

"I can't spend two nights in the hospital," she told the doctor when he first issued the directive. "I have three other children at home to take care of."

"All my patients stay that long."

"Are you sure?" She wanted to believe him.

"Relax. You had two successful deliveries, one with twins. The odds are in your favor." The doctor's tone left her feeling more anxious, but nothing she said changed his mind.

She walks through the house calling Rick's name, then grabs the car keys. When she pushes open the garage door, he looks up from the workbench where he's sorting mail.

"You're doing that now?" Her voice is stretched tight. "We're going to be late."

He laughs. "I've been waiting for you."

Say nothing, she instructs herself silently. *Unless you want to drive yourself.*

Rick follows her outside. "You know," he says playfully. "My father once told me a happy wife makes for a happy life."

"Oh yeah?" She stifles a laugh. "When am I going to see that?" She turns to hide her broad smile. The truth is, she's happy and he knows it. Yet, as he drives through the neighborhood, a parade of concerns march through her head, the ones her OBGYN dismissed each time she asked.

"You're not too old at forty-one," the doctor said. "It's not too soon after your last delivery. Yes, it's safe to have another Caesarian." When Marianne persisted with questions, he held up his hand like a crossing guard. "You worry too much."

Her shoulders slumped. "I can't help it. My mother worries. Her mother worried. It's in my DNA."

"Women have been having babies for centuries," the doctor said. "You're no different."

If you only knew. I've felt different all my life, even before my father died. I never fit in or felt comfortable in my own skin. Her uncles called her weird, her brothers said she was adopted, and her mother started her on a diet when she turned eight. *I never felt normal.* Certain he wouldn't understand, she didn't bother to explain. Instead, she trusted the doctor's advice.

"We're here." Rick pulls into the hospital lot. Marianne turns to face him, happy in the moment.

"I can't wait to meet our son."

In the delivery room, the doctor's hands work behind a cloth drape like a magician.

"Everything's fine," he says. "You can stop crying." The doctor gives a reassuring look. She wants to stop, but the tears don't let up. "See?" He lifts the newborn. "Your son is perfect." He moves towards the nurse. "Show her, please."

She places the newborn on Marianne's chest. *What a miracle you are.* Marianne presses her face into his black curls.

"I count ten fingers and ten toes," Rick says.

She inhales the baby's scent. "Thank God."

"He looks like me; good looks run on my side."

"You wish." A smile lifts the corners of her mouth.

"I'll get him cleaned up," the nurse says. As she carries the baby away, Marianne panics.

"Go follow our baby," she tells Rick.

He moves fast on her order, trailing the nurse to the weighing station while Marianne is wheeled to recovery where she calls home. The twins answer on the first ring.

"Hi, Mom." Their voices trace each other. "How's our new baby brother doing?"

"He's absolutely gorgeous. Wait till you see his long eyelashes. How are you?"

"We're fine," Britney says.

"Is Grandma there?"

"Yeah, right here," Amber says.

"Marianne?" Vera's voice sounds strained.

"Ma? You okay?"

"That's what I want to ask you."

"I'm good, Ma."

"Thank God. And the baby? How's the baby?"

"He's perfect."

"I can't tell you how much I prayed."

"Me too." The nurse walks in with the baby. "I have to go, Ma. John looks hungry." The nurse passes Marianne the baby and a bottle.

"He's big for a preemie," she says.

"John takes after my father. He was over six feet." Marianne studies her son: his skin, tan like hers, his turned-up nose, and his long, delicate fingers like a musician. She imagines an older version of John, standing at a keyboard, playing music. She holds the bottle for him like she did with her other babies and waits for him to latch on to the nipple. Instead, he stares at her with his mouth open.

"He's not liking this," she tells the nurse. Milk dribbles down his cheek. "Can we try a different bottle?"

The nurse moves in close. "It's all in the technique." She wedges a pillow underneath Marianne's elbow. "Don't worry, he'll figure it out. I'll be back." Marianne moves the bottle the way the nurse did.

"Take your time, John. I'm not going anywhere."

He stares at her face.

"Your brother and sisters are going to love you. Your father, too. I'll have to stand in line." She tells him about her favorite beach at the Jersey Shore and how the boardwalk lights up at night. As she describes the rushing ocean waves toppling over her, the hot sand stinging her feet, and the almond scent of suntan oil, she loses herself in the memory. "We will have so much fun together."

When he finally drinks from the bottle, he guzzles four ounces. *That nurse was right.* Happy John got the hang of it, Marianne dozes with him in her arms.

John wakes up like clockwork his first night, filling his belly every four hours. She doesn't remember her other kids being this hungry. When John is not eating, he sinks into a deep, unmoving slumber. The next day, he is circumcised like his brother was two years earlier. That's where the similarities end.

"John was the best patient ever," the nurse brags after the procedure. "He didn't cry or make a fuss."

Rick chuckles. "I remember how Robby woke up the entire hospital wing." He looks at Marianne. "I guess John is going to be the easy one."

"Thank God for that."

Before the sun is up on the third day, Marianne is packed and ready to go home. When the nurse arrives with a wheelchair, she brushes it off.

""Sorry. Everyone gets a ride." The nurse puts a small photograph into Marianne's hand. "This was taken just a few minutes after his birth." She cradles the photo like a chalice. In the picture, her son stares straight into the camera, his eyes alert, his lips set in a straight line, and his tiny fists snug to his face like a boxer ready for a fight.

"Oh my," Marianne sighs, head over heels in love.

At home, she carries John around the house while Robby walks alongside holding her hand. They sit together in the warm August sun, watching the girls play with friends. *Amber, Britney, Robby, and John. I am so happy to be your mother.* In college, when sorority sisters swapped news of job offers, Marianne stuffed a pillow under her sweatshirt.

"This is the job I want."

That evening, they all sit together in the kitchen while Vera cooks dinner. As she stirs spaghetti in the boiling water, the aroma of garlic and onions rises from the back burner.

"Hurry up with the food, Ma. I'm starving."

Vera lifts the wooden spoon from the pot. "Don't push it." Marianne laughs, though not entirely sure if her mother is kidding. At seventy-eight, Vera is full of surprises. Rick sniffs the air as he walks in.

"That smells good."

"Isn't my mother unbelievable?" Marianne says. "Come on girls. Let's set the table."

I didn't expect to remarry after my first marriage ended, not with two little girls to care for, until I had a reading with a famous Long Island psychic. She knew my first name had two n's, which no one gets right, so I was impressed from the start. She also knew I didn't have a man in my life but said things were about to change. 'You will marry a man named Rick and have two more children,' she said. From then on, I had my eyes open for someone named Rick.

One summer weekend when my girlfriends and I went to the Parker House at the Jersey Shore, I saw a cute guy sitting at the bar watching baseball.

'Who's winning?' I asked.

He shrugged.

'What's your name?'

I thought I heard him say 'Greg,' but the music was too loud to talk. He was there again the next time we went.

'Hi Greg,' I said. 'Wanna dance?'

'My name's not Greg. It's Rick.'

I ran over to my girlfriends and jumped up and down.

'His name is Rick! His name is Rick!'

He was seven years younger, which didn't bother him at all. He also liked the idea of a ready-made family and wanted two more children once we were married.

'You picked the right girl for that,' I told him. All my life, I wanted four children. So, after we had Robby, we had one more. We both have the same values when it comes to family. (Marianne)

ONE MONTH OLD

BEST LIFE EVER

Marianne dresses John for his first public outing in early September. "It's my cousin's annual Labor Day barbecue," she tells him. "Everyone will be there -- aunts, uncles, and cousins. They can't wait to meet you and I can't wait to show you off."

"The car is packed," Rick says. "Vera and the kids are outside. We're ready to go."

"Five minutes," she says.

He looks down at her pajamas. "Seriously?"

"Okay. Ten."

A few minutes later, she buckles John into the car seat. In the back, the girls bicker over who will sit next to Grandma.

"One on either side." Vera scooches over to make room. Robby reaches for his brother's hand.

"Oh, Robby, your brother is sleeping. You can play when he wakes up." Marianne settles into the passenger seat.

"We're going to be late," Rick says. "It's a holiday weekend, so there'll be bumper-to-bumper traffic." He speeds through the neighborhood. "We should've left earlier."

"Don't be such a Danny Downer. No one cares what time we get there. They only want to meet John."

Rick inches the car onto the crowded highway. "I wish I brought coffee."

"Here, have mine."

He takes a sip, then grimaces. "It's cold."

"It's the thought that counts." When he doesn't smile, she tries another tack. "Okay, admit it: you won't be happy until you're drinking a beer with the guys."

Rick shrugs. "You say that like it's a bad thing." As the car idles in highway traffic, he fiddles with the air conditioning, then rolls down his window. Marianne doesn't mind the traffic or the heat. There's no other place she'd rather be. She looks around at her mother, the kids, and Rick. *This is my tribe. It doesn't get much better than this.*

They arrive at the barbeque with the sun low in the sky. People cheer when they see John and scurry to get close. Amber and Britney run off with Robby to find their cousins, while Rick heads to the grill, where he's handed a bottle of beer and a burger. Vera reaches for John, then calls out to her sister, Anna, and her sisters-in-law, Annie and Flo.

"Come meet my grandson." The women sit in chairs against a fence and pass John among themselves. In the dimming light, Rick snaps a dozen pictures with his new camera: a self-portrait with Robby, Marianne with the girls and Robby, and all of them with John. After each shot, Marianne shuts her eyes, hoping to imprint the memory of how full her heart feels.

That night at home, she helps the girls get ready for bed, while Rick takes charge of the boys. When the house is quiet, he sits alert in bed. She senses he has something to say, but she is too bone-tired for a conversation.

"I want to talk about John."

She wants to drift off to sleep listening to the sound of her son's name.

"It's important," Rick says. She sits up to listen. "I've been a hands-on father since day one, right? I changed Robby's diapers, gave him baths, and got up in the middle of the night to feed him.

And now, I do that with John. Am I right?"

"Yes, you're right. Can we go to sleep now?"

"John is different from Robby."

"Every one of our children is different. Even Amber and Britney are as different as night and day."

"That's not what I mean. When I change Robby into his pajamas, he kicks and pushes me away. John doesn't move like that. He hardly moves at all."

"Can we talk about this tomorrow?"

"I think there's something wrong with John."

His words land with a hard blow. "Are you nuts?"

"He's asleep when I leave for work in the morning and asleep when I get home. On weekends, he sleeps all the time."

"One day you'll wish he would take a nap so you can get some rest."

"I want a doctor to check him out."

"That's crazy."

"I'm not giving up on this." He turns off the light. As his breathing slows to a rhythm, Marianne tries to quiet the worry that gnaws at her. Of course, she noticed how much John sleeps and was concerned enough to ask her mother about it.

"Don't worry," Vera told her. "He drinks milk, he's chubby; he's a good baby."

Tonight, though, those reassurances are no match for Rick's words. There's something wrong with John. Her heart burns with fear as the morning sun blazes through the window.

Rick picks up the conversation the next morning as soon as he sees her in the kitchen. "The way John is, it's not normal."

"What's not normal?" Vera says as she fills the espresso pot with coffee.

"I think there's something wrong with John."

"That's ridiculous," Vera says.

Marianne raises her eyebrows at Rick. *I told you so.*

"All I know is that when I carry him, it's like trying to hold on to Jell-O. It's not normal."

"Stop talking like that." Vera slaps a dishtowel in the air, then storms out.

"See what you did."

"I'm sure your mother noticed the same things."

"Fine. Why don't you come to John's next wellness exam? Ask the doctor yourself."

Later in the day, one of her cousins calls to apologize for missing the barbeque.

"I hear your son is gorgeous." Her cousin's voice is soft and dreamy. "Aren't newborns wonderful?"

"Especially mine. John is either the best baby in the world or there's something wrong." Marianne is surprised to hear herself repeat Rick's words.

"Don't say that. I'm sure your son is perfect."

"You're right. You're so right." Marianne backtracks fast. "I'm such a worry-wart."

On the first day of seventh grade, the twins' father passes away. He was sick, but his death is unexpected.

"I'm so sorry," Marianne tells her daughters.

"We saw him last weekend," Britney says. "He was fine."

"Your father always felt good when you were with him. He loved you very much."

"I can't believe we won't see him again."

When her own father died, Marianne was two years younger than her daughters. That last time, he was dressing up for a night on the town with his wife and his in-laws.

"Who's the most handsome daddy in the world?" he asked her, smiling.

"You are." She reached up to fix his bow tie.

At the restaurant, her father said he didn't feel good and stepped outside for air. In three short bursts, he had one heart attack after another. Her uncles carried him across the street to the Emergency Room, but her father didn't make it. No one understood how a forty-seven-year-old man died so fast.

At school, Marianne was "the sad girl with no father." Her Uncle Danny escorted her to the father-daughter dance so she wouldn't be left out. She smiles at the memory of him in his favorite brown suit and fancy shoes. He twirled her on the dance floor, and they won first prize. When Uncle Danny died, Marianne lost a father for a second time.

"You can cry all you want," she tells her daughters. "Your sisters are sad," she tells the boys. "Let's show them some love." Robby climbs into the twins' laps, one then the other, and hugs them. They take turns holding John.

When Rick arrives home, he sits with them. "I liked your dad," he says. Marianne remembers when the two men walked together on the boardwalk at the Jersey Shore, talking about who-knows-what, back when the girls were in grade school and Robby was a baby. Her ex-husband carried Robby while Rick held the twins' hands, and she wondered how she got so lucky.

The next day, she tries again with the twins. "I'm here if you want to talk or you can go to a counselor. Whichever is better for you." The girls agree to one session but don't want more.

"It's a waste of time," Amber says.

Britney agrees. "There's nothing to talk about."

Marianne doesn't push, though she wants to; anything to prevent them from stuffing their feelings down inside the way she did. The girls will return to school in a few days like nothing's wrong, but their lives are forever changed. She knows how it feels and how long it lasts.

"Your son is taller and weighs more than ninety percent of children in his age group," the pediatrician says at John's wellness exam. When he offers his finger to John, the baby grabs hold. "How is his eating?"

"He spits up formula like his brother did," Marianne says. "Can we try the lighter formula we used with Robby?"

"Of course." The doctor hands her a prescription. "Anything else?"

Marianne gives Rick a look.

"John sleeps all the time," Rick says. "And when I hold him, it feels like he's about to slip out of my hands. It's not normal."

She winces at the word.

"I don't see anything to worry about."

Rick looks unsettled. "Are you sure?"

"As sure as I can be, but if you want peace of mind, take him to this doctor." He hands Rick a business card. "He's one of the best pediatric neurologists. He can tell you what's wrong, if anything is." Later that day, Marianne books an appointment.

"One problem," she tells Rick. "The earliest they can see him is two-weeks out."

"Two weeks? We can't wait that long. Can you ask Patti if she can get us an earlier appointment? She works with doctors, right? She has contacts."

"I hate to ask."

"She's your friend since college. And, you're not asking for yourself; you're asking for John. You know she'd want to help."

The next day, Marianne reaches out.

"You were right to ask," Patti says. "I'll see what I can do." Early the next day, she calls back. "John has an appointment tomorrow if you want it. The doctor is a New York specialist with a second office in New Jersey, he's twenty minutes from you."

"Is he any good?" Marianne says.

"All the doctors I work with say he's an expert."

That night, Marianne paces the kitchen.

"What's wrong?" Vera says. She picks at a piece of Entenmann's crumb cake.

"John needs to see a specialist. A pediatric neurologist."

"Did you tell your brother?"

"Robert's a psychiatrist, Ma. He doesn't know about this."

Vera dials her son's number. "Robert? Your sister needs to speak with you." She passes Marianne the phone.

"Hi, Robert. I'm sorry to bother you." She tells him about the referral from the doctor.

"Sounds like you should take John," he says. "Do you want me to come?"

"No, I'm sure it's nothing." Her heart pounds against her chest, despite her casual tone.

The next morning, while she and Rick try to get comfortable in the doctor's waiting room, her head spins with worry. *What if something is wrong? How will we handle that?* She steals a glance at the others waiting with them: a boy she guesses to be about eleven or twelve, in a wheelchair, and a woman she imagines is his mother. The boy makes sounds, but speaks no words. He flaps his arms like bird wings. He is trying to say something, that much is clear. The woman leans in close and listens. Marianne looks away, embarrassed to stare. *That poor boy. That poor mother. I could never deal with that.*

The nurse leads them to an exam room where the doctor introduces himself. He listens to John's lungs and heart, stretches the baby's arms and legs, and turns him onto his belly. The doctor's examination lasts more than twenty minutes.

"Can you feed him?" he says.

Marianne holds John and sends him mental messages. *You can do this.* She slides the nipple into his mouth. *You got this.* Almost instantly, John drinks from the bottle.

"I've seen enough," the doctor says. "Your son has what's called hypermobility. That means his arms and legs stretch further than most babies."

"My two sisters are double-jointed," Rick says. "Could John have that?"

"Maybe. Double-jointed children often look floppy at this age." The doctor hands Rick a sheet of paper with stick figures in various poses. "Do these exercises with him every day. They will help him get stronger." He closes the file. "I wouldn't worry. Your son will catch up by the time he's three."

After the appointment, Marianne and Rick sit in the car while John sleeps in his car seat.

"I'm relieved," Rick says. "I was positive there was something wrong."

"You had me convinced. Deep down, I was terrified."

"Looks like we worried for nothing," he says.

"Thank God. I can handle anything except if one of our kids gets sick."

"Let's tell our parents the good news."

After the specialist said John was fine, we all relaxed. My mother moved back to the duplex in Yonkers she shared with her older sister, the twins invited friends for sleepovers, and Robby doted on his little brother more than before. Rick focused on building his business and I was happy at home. Sure, John's medical scare detoured us, but we stepped back into our lives once he was in the clear. (Marianne)

TWO MONTHS OLD

SHOCK WAVES

One autumn afternoon, a new message flashes on the answering machine. Marianne listens to the unfamiliar voice.

"I'm calling to remind you of John's appointment at ten a.m. tomorrow." Then she remembers: it's the neurologist his pediatrician recommended.

"I forgot to cancel," she tells Rick.

"John doesn't need another appointment. We already know he's fine."

"I don't want his pediatrician to think we're rude."

"Want me to come?"

"No, it will be a quick. I'm sure we'll be home in no time."

That night, John sits in the plastic baby tub in the sink. He smiles as she splashes him with warm water. "Wait till I take you to the ocean with Robby and your sisters. Daddy will come, too." John rests his head against her hand until the water chills.

He sleeps later than usual in the morning, and waking him is difficult. As she dresses him, Marianne has an ominous feeling about the day. She wishes she had canceled as Rick suggested. Of all the times she should have listened, this tops the list.

At the doctor's office, she forces herself to sit. *Calm down. We know there's nothing wrong with John.* But the knot in her stomach tightens.

"We're ready for you," the nurse says. In the exam room the doctor asks no questions. Instead, he lays John on the table and watches him breathe.

"I'll be right back," the doctor says. As he walks out, a shiver runs through her.

"What a silly man." Her cheery voice disguises her racing heart. She wants to run out of the room with John, but the doctor returns with another man.

"This is my business partner; I'd like his opinion." The two men move around the exam table looking at John as though he is a lab specimen.

"What do you think?" the first doctor asks.

"He definitely has it."

"I agree. In fact, I'm sure of it."

The partner nods at Marianne. "Good luck." He closes the door behind him.

"You can dress him," the doctor says.

Finally. She is grateful to be done with this.

"Is your husband with you?" the doctor asks.

"My husband? No, he's at work."

"Can we get him here?"

"Why? What's wrong?"

"We can't be sure without a DNA test."

"DNA? What are you talking about?"

"Let's talk more in my office."

Her legs don't move.

"Here, let me take the baby," he says. She passes John with shaky hands. *I've got to get control of myself.* The doctor leads her to a cluttered office, and points to a chair across from his desk.

"I can hold him now." Marianne takes a deep breath. "Please tell me."

"You need a test to confirm the diagnosis, but we think he has something called SMA."

How bad can three letters be?

"SMA stands for Spinal Muscular Atrophy. It's the most common genetic cause of infant death."

"If you think my son has a genetic disease, you couldn't be more wrong. I had genetic testing before I got pregnant and so did my husband. After I was pregnant, I had a sonogram and amniocentesis; those results were normal, too. No one said anything about this disease."

"You need to ask to be tested."

"I never heard of it. How would I know to ask?"

"You wouldn't, unfortunately."

"How did John get it?"

"Both parents must carry the defective gene. Then, when a carrier has a child with another carrier, there is a one-in-four chance their child will have SMA."

How do I tell Rick it's our fault?

"Do you have other children?"

"Twin daughters who are almost twelve. Another son, almost two."

"They all should be tested."

Her head spins with all this information.

"Have you heard of ALS?" the doctor says.

"Lou Gehrig's disease?"

"That's another name for it."

"What does that have to do with John?"

"SMA is sometimes called Infantile ALS. They are both neuromuscular diseases."

"What happens with SMA?"

The doctor uses strange words like "autosomal," "recessive," and "motor neurons." She wishes she had concentrated more in science classes. "Ordinarily, the brain sends instructions to the muscles and when received, the muscles move as the brain instructs. With SMA, the body is missing the motor neurons that are needed to send the messages."

She stares at the doctor's face; never before has she understood so little.

"Because the muscles don't receive the messages, they eventually atrophy. Most children with SMA don't make it to their second birthday."

"What? That's preposterous." Her heart pounds against her chest. "Did you bother to read the report the specialist faxed?"

"Actually, that doctor also suspected SMA."

"No. No way." Marianne shakes her head furiously. "He said we had nothing to worry about." Her memory is clear.

"Hypermobility, he called it. He said John would outgrow it by age three. He was certain."

"It's in his notes." The doctor points to a highlighted sentence and reads. "If no improvement within three months, test for SMA." He passes her the file. "See for yourself." She wants to scream, but now's not the time.

"How can we help John?"

"It would be better if he had cancer than this. At least with cancer, there are treatments and sometimes a cure. With SMA, there's nothing."

"I have to get my son home." She struggles to stand.

"You can stay until you feel better."

Unless this is a joke, I will never feel better. She clutches John to her chest and moves her feet. Every step is deliberate. She walks out of the building and looks for the car. She straps John into his seat. Three times she dials a wrong number. Finally, on the fourth try she gets Rick.

"Hello?"

She can't seem to speak the words.

"Marianne, what's wrong? What happened?"

"The doctor says John has a disease called SMA."

"What?"

"SMA. A genetic disease."

"That can't be."

"He said we will lose our son before he's two years old." The words spill out of her.

"Let me look it up." He quickly taps the keyboard. "Did he take any blood?"

"No."

"Did you tell him about the expert who saw John?"

"That doctor saw the same disease. I saw his file."

"Impossible. He would've said something."

"We can't lose him, Rick. We haven't even gotten to know him yet."

"Don't listen to that quack. He had no right to scare you."

"You should've seen his face. He was so certain."

At home, she looks for Rick as soon as John is asleep. "Did you call that other doctor?"

Rick nods.

"And?"

"He said he wasn't sure because John's legs were stronger than his arms, which he typically doesn't see with SMA. He didn't say anything because he didn't want to worry us."

"That wasn't his call. He had no right."

"He apologized," Rick says.

"Did you tell him not to bother?"

"He offered to help decipher the DNA results."

"As if we'd want his help."

"We might. We should keep our options open."

The next day, the children have their blood drawn at a nearby laboratory.

"Results take two weeks or longer," the tech says.

"Two weeks?" Marianne looks at Rick. "How will we ever last that long?"

That night, he sits at the computer, researching.

"Find anything?" she asks.

"Nothing I understand. I'll ask my sister, Laurie, for help. She talks to doctors on her job, so she knows the medical jargon."

"Tell her thanks for me. I'm happy for the help."

"Is John going to die?" Britney says the next morning.

Marianne tries to answer the question without adding her own fears to the mix.

"We hope not. He has good doctors."

"Losing dad was bad enough," Amber says. "We can't lose anyone else we love."

"I don't want to lose him either," Marianne says.

"How can we help?"

"You are good sisters. He's lucky to have you. For now, try not to worry."

I was so ignorant. I thought everything bad would have been identified through prenatal testing. Never in my wildest imagination did I think a terminal disease like Spinal Muscular Atrophy would slip by untested. (Marianne)

I was hell-bent on proving the expert wrong. When I got down deep into the medical articles, though, I thought my head would explode; it was like reading a foreign language. I read the same paragraphs six, seven, eight times, trying to understand. (Rick)

THREE MONTHS OLD

FREE FALLING

"I've got to do something," she tells Karen, her best friend since college.

"You take care of your children, your husband, and your home," Karen says. "It's not like you do nothing."

"You know what I mean. This thing with John."

"About that.... Do you believe in faith healers?"

"I believe in anything that helps John."

"A famous healer is coming to New York City this weekend. We can take John."

"Let's do it. We have nothing to lose."

On Saturday, Karen leads the way through the crowds that

pack the street. "Please let us through," she says in a loud voice. "We're trying to save this child." The crowd opens, allowing them to pass. The church stairs are packed, too, but Karen moves them up with ease. Once inside, she moves them through the throng of people to the front of the church.

The faith healer invites them to come closer. Marianne holds John in extended arms as the holy man prays. Afterwards, Marianne can't wait to talk with Karen.

"Do you think there was a healing? It sure felt like it to me."

"Me too," Karen says. "The question is, who was healed?"

"I hope it's John. That's why we came all this way." Her stomach grumbles. "If I'm hungry, he must be famished. Where I can feed him?"

A churchwoman taps her gently on the arm. "There's an empty room downstairs."

Marianne follows Karen to a dark auditorium. They sit on the bleachers while Marianne feeds John.

"I smell something good."

"Me too," Karen says."

"I have to find out what it is." She passes the baby to Karen and walks to the other side of the room. "It's bread and still warm." She carries the loaf to Karen. "Do you think it's sacrilegious if we eat some?" Without waiting for an answer, Marianne pulls off a piece. "Oh, Karen. This is the most delicious bread I've ever tasted."

"Maybe it's Miracle Bread," Karen says.

"Miracle Bread? Oh my God, maybe it is." She rubs a piece on John's head. "Miracle Bread, Miracle Bread," she chants. Suddenly, a woman appears next to Marianne.

"This was my daughter's Rosary." She pours a string of crystal beads into Marianne's hand. "They will help your son." The woman quickly disappears as if she never existed.

"Do you think she was an apparition?" Marianne says.

"We both saw her," Karen says.

"Where did she come from?"

"Maybe she's an angel sent to help John." Karen smiles, her mouth full of bread.

During the next week, a Catholic priest blesses John with Holy Water, a minister lays hands on him, and a clairvoyant clears his aura.

"I'm trying everything," Marianne tells Rick. "Who knows what will help."

"I want to take him to one more doctor," he says.

"I'm too exhausted for another appointment. You'll have

to go without me."

"Robert said he'd come."

"You called my brother?"

"To ask if he learned about SMA in medical school."

"What did he say?"

"He never heard of the disease."

Later that night while the others sleep, Marianne sits holding John, stunned by the beauty of his face. *You certainly don't look like a sick child.*

The next afternoon, Rick returns from the doctor's appointment looking deflated.

"How did it go?" Marianne lifts John from the car seat and buries her face in his neck.

"I told her how that doctor scared you," Rick says. "She said he was her mentor and was very smart."

"I'm sorry I wasn't there."

"Then, she examined John and said, 'I can't tell you what you want to hear. You need to wait for the test results.' In the elevator afterwards, I think your brother was crying."

Deep down, Marianne's not surprised. A part of her knows John has this disease and from the way he looks at her, John knows it too.

"You are more gorgeous than ever," she tells him. His hair is longer, with waves and curls. He gives her an impish smile. Do you understand what's happening?"

John's eyes lock on hers, unblinking. He holds her gaze, and in that moment she has her answer: he understands, and is ready for the fight of his life.

On the day the DNA results are due, the family sits together, waiting for the phone to ring. The twins have homework, Robby needs a nap, Marianne has housework, and Rick should be at the office, but no one leaves. The phone rings all day, with her mother and brothers wanting to know the test results. When Vera calls again, Rick takes the phone.

"Can you ask everyone to stop," Rick says. "We have to keep the line open for the doctor." He promises to call as soon as they know. When the phone rings at five o'clock, Marianne is sure it's the doctor.

"You answer," she tells Rick. "I just can't do it."

He picks up the phone and listens to the doctor, Marianne scanning his face for clues. He hangs up the phone and looks at his family. It's the saddest face she's ever seen.

"It's positive. John has SMA."

Marianne collapses into the chair, her body folding in on

itself. The girls throw their arms around her. Robby hugs her. Rick stands in front of them all, his jaw set in determination.

"We will beat this," he says. "We will."

There are no words to describe how I felt to hear the terminal diagnosis. I experienced grief before -- my father died, my ex-husband died, my favorite uncle died, but with John, this was much more than anything I knew. (Marianne)

After John's diagnosis was confirmed, my research shifted to finding out if there was a cure in play for SMA. Yet despite what I knew, I bought a tiny reflex hammer after reading that children with SMA have no reflexes. I must have tapped John's knee a hundred thousand times, looking for movement, figuring if he had a reflex, he didn't have the disease. (Rick)

FOUR MONTHS OLD

LIVES ON THE LINE

Marianne is inconsolable. Nothing anyone says brings comfort. How can she go on with life if they lose him?

"If John goes, I will go too," Marianne tells Rick. "You stay with the girls and Robby."

"What? No, you can't do that."

"You are good with them."

"The children need you."

"Then we all go with John." She imagines an earthquake or hurricane taking them all out.

"No. Just no."

She misses her father. If he were here, he'd know what to

do. She needs him now more than ever.

Vera moves back in, with more suitcases than before. Rick sets up an office in the house, and Marianne spends time with the children in John's room.

"We must show him how much he is loved. It's the only thing that matters."

Laurie's research becomes more urgent as they race to beat the clock. She calls one night with an update. "SMA is a niche disease with very few experts. Most doctors never heard of it, and many of the neurologists I spoke with had heard the name but nothing more."

"Is there anyone?" Rick says.

"There is a pediatric neurologist in Maryland who has examined more than a hundred children with SMA. He can see John if you want an appointment."

This time when Robert offers to go with them, Marianne accepts. "Maybe you can decipher the medical information."

"Don't count on it. I know as little as you."

On the drive to Baltimore, John coos and smiles, not at all in pain. She cannot fathom the idea that she will lose him in just a few short months.

At the office, the doctor smiles with confidence.

"We hope you can show us how to help our son," Rick says.

The doctor listens to John's heartbeat and his lungs. He flexes John's arms and his legs. The doctor takes measurements and jots notes in a medical file.

"I agree with the other doctors. Your son has SMA. Probably SMA1 because he is so young. It's one of the worst."

Marianne is too stunned to speak.

"Most babies with SMA1 don't live past six months." The doctor pulls a pie chart from his file cabinet. "Ninety percent died within the first six months of diagnosis," he points to the largest piece of the pie.

Marianne struggles to find her breath.

"Another five percent died before age one." He points to a narrow slice.

Inhale, two, three, four. Hold. Exhale, two, three, four.

"Only five percent reached their second birthday." He points to the smallest sliver of the pie. "Unfortunately, they were diagnosed much older than your son."

"There must be something we can do?" she says.

"Water therapy is the number one thing that helps. Most babies find warm water soothing."

"What else?" Rick says.

"Beyond that, there is really nothing."

"How can there be nothing? There are advances in science and medicine every day."

"I'm afraid there is good news and bad news when it comes to SMA research."

"What's the good news?" Marianne allows for the briefest moment of hope.

"SMA is the number one most curable neuromuscular disease today."

"The bad news?"

"There won't be a treatment or cure for at least ten to fifteen years. Your son won't live long enough."

She wants to cover John's ears. The voice inside her screams to block out this news. The room feels like it's shrinking.

The doctor's predictions preoccupy her during the ride home. She cradles John in the back seat, unwilling to let go. That night, she sits alone in the kitchen as the last glow of daylight slips away. She has no idea how to live with such a cataclysmic tragedy.

She moves through the days, numb. Thoughts of losing John consume her. She doesn't eat, doesn't sleep, and doesn't want to go on living. Yet, she knows something has to change. The children all deserve happy childhoods, and it's up to her to help them make good memories. *How can I help them if I can't help myself?* How can she save John if she can't save herself?

At John's next appointment, the pediatrician hands her a folder of information about SMA.

"You don't have to do this alone," he says. "Your school district has special services called Early Intervention. John can receive at-home teaching and other services." He scribbles a name on his prescription pad. "I also know an excellent physical therapist whose name is Rashida. I'm sure she can help him."

In late October, the twins corner her one night.

"Mom, we want to go Trick or Treating on Halloween," Amber tells her.

"And dress up as princesses," Britney chimes in.

Wanting things to be as normal as possible, Marianne helps them pick out costumes. On Halloween, she dresses Robby as Winnie the Pooh and John as his faithful companion, Tigger.

"Didn't Robby wear that last year?" Rick asks.

"Yes, but his costume goes with John's outfit."

"Marianne, can't you see he's outgrown it?" Rick sounds annoyed in a way she's not used to. She realizes the Tigger costume is not really the problem; when your child has a life-threatening disease, matching costumes is the least important thing.

"This is the last year Robby wears that costume," she tells Rick. "I promise."

In early November, Rashida arranges to visit John at home. The night she arrives, she watches John receive laser treatment.

"It's supposed to help his motor neurons." Marianne glides a wand along John's back.

"What a beautiful baby," Rashida says.

"Do you work with babies as sick as my son?"

"I work with all babies."

"Do you know anything about SMA?"

"I know a little."

"The doctors say there is no hope."

"Doctors don't know everything," Rashida says. "May I hold him?" As she places John on the floor, he smiles. "The big thing is to keep him moving." She rolls John onto one side and then the other. She massages his hands and feet. She lays him on his belly. "To improve his flexibility and strength, he's got to keep moving." John seems to relax with her easy way.

"I can help your son," Rashida says. "My schedule is full so I can only come at night. Is that good for you?"

"Nobody goes to sleep early in this house. Any time before

one in the morning works fine."

"If we take it slow, he will get stronger. You will see."

The next day Marianne calls Rashida. "My mother says John looks better today than he did yesterday. Whatever you did helped him. Thank you."

"I'm happy to hear this. I look forward to working with him in the new year."

That night, as Marianne bathes John, she moves his legs in the water. "The important thing is to keep you moving. We are very lucky to have found Rashida."

For the Thanksgiving holiday, Marianne invites Rick's parents, his sisters and their families, and her two brothers and their families for holiday dinner. A few days before the event, she wants to cancel.

"What was I thinking?" she asks her mother.

"Don't worry," Vera says. "I'll help." She bakes lasagna as a first course while Rick prepares turkey and stuffing. The girls make yams and cranberry sauce. Marianne helps them bake a pumpkin pie for dessert.

Everyone arrives hungry. John sleeps in her arms as plates of food are passed around. Marianne marvels at how normal it seems until she remembers he has a few months left. There's nothing normal in that.

In December, the house feels like a funeral parlor waiting for the corpse to arrive. She avoids the calendar. She forces her feet to move. She reminds herself to breathe. She's not the only one trying to make it. Rick walks around without a word; the girls want to stay home; Robby clings.

"We want a Christmas tree," Britney says one day.

Amber agrees. "With presents underneath."

"The kids want to celebrate Christmas," she tells Rick. "They deserve to, don't they?"

He brings home a tree as high as the ceiling. The girls hang tinsel; Robby and Rick hang ornaments. Marianne summons energy she doesn't know is there.

"I'm going to take the kids to the Mall for pictures with Santa," she tells Robert.

"I'm not sure that's a good idea," he says. "We don't know enough to risk an infection or the flu."

Instead, she buys a life-sized plastic Santa who sings holiday music at the press of a button. The girls, dressed in red and green holiday outfits, pose in front of him. The boys, wearing matching colors, sit with their sisters, one in each lap. Rick focuses his camera.

"No one's smiling," he says. "I can't get a good picture if no one smiles."

When she looks at the children, she sees the weight of their sadness. She is sure they see that same sadness on her face. If they are to feel joy even as their brother is sick, she has to show them it's okay. If they are to have a happy childhood in the middle of these terrible circumstances, she has to give it to them. She can start by smiling. They have to see that it's okay to smile. It's okay to be happy. It's okay to play. It's up to her to show them.

She imagines herself on the beach with all of them, soaking up sun, splashing in the waves. Steeped in memory, she smiles. Like magic, the girls smile; Robby laughs.

"Say cheese," Rick says. He takes the shot and then a dozen more just to make sure he has the best one.

The week between Christmas and New Year's moves fast. She keeps the children close and keeps all of them close to John. She's grateful no one asks too much of her. Statistics gives them two more months with John. She can't believe they will lose him, no matter how hard she tries. He gurgles, giggles, and laughs like any other baby.

On New Year's Eve, Rick comes home with champagne. "It's a gift from one of my clients." He pours each of them a glass.

"What's to celebrate?" Marianne says.

"We're together. That's something."

"It's amazing how I put up with you." She's surprised by her own humor.

"I think the doctors are wrong," Rick says with bravado.

"What do you mean?"

"What if he can live long enough for the cure?"

"Do you think it's possible?"

"Why not?"

Marianne remembers Karen's favorite expression: if we can see it, it can happen.

"Let's start a tradition," Rick says. "Each year that John is with us, we'll save the champagne bottle as a reminder of how far he's come."

"I'm in. Maybe we really can turn this thing around."

If you make a list of every expert involved in SMA research at the time, I probably had a personal conversation with each of them. Marianne's sister-in-law who's fluent in French helped us talk to a doctor in Paris. I spoke to doctors all around the world. They all had ideas but said it's at least a ten to fifteen-year wait before any treatment hits the market. (Rick)

Everyone in my office worked to find the people who held the keys to the research kingdom. One doctor gave us hope. 'Don't take anything at face value,' he said. 'The diagnosis is not a fait accompli.' But he was the only one. We felt lost but kept at it because we were trying to save John's life. When it's a purpose above self, you have energy and confidence but there was another force, a God-force that gave us extra strength to work non-stop. (Laurie, Rick's sister)

FIVE MONTHS OLD

PUSH THE EDGES

As the end of time stampedes towards them, Marianne shrinks the house to one small corner near John's room. She drags a couch, a few chairs, and a folding table. The girls do homework near John and bring friends over to visit. Robby reads his picture books to John. Marianne keeps vigil, watching them all and helping where she can. Rick casts a wider net for SMA treatments.

"We want cutting-edge technology," he tells his sister.

"I found one doctor who claims to clone children without disease," Laurie says.

Marianne contacts the doctor the next day.

"Yes," he says. "I can help you."

"How does it work?"

"From the mother, I take a good egg and create a healthy embryo. Nine months later, you have a clone."

She tries to picture it. "Are you telling us that there will be two Johns?"

"Yes, of course."

"How does that help our son?"

"My dear, cloning creates a second child who does not have the disease but is otherwise the same child you have now."

"Then what happens to John?"

"He will be taken by the disease eventually."

"We're trying to save our son, doctor. Not create a new one." She can't wait to hang up.

"That guy was no help," she tells Rick that night. "Most of it sounded like science fiction."

"I have another lead not as far-fetched. Stem cells."

"Stem cells?"

"A doctor in Atlanta transplants stem cells into his ALS patients. SMA is called infantile ALS. So, if stem cells can help ALS patients, maybe they can help John." The next morning, Marianne calls the Atlanta doctor.

"I'm sorry," he says. "I only treat adults."

"But ALS is similar to SMA."

"The way you describe SMA, yes, there are similarities."

"Then your treatment should work for John."

"Something could go wrong," the doctor says.

"My husband and I will sign whatever you need. We think it's worth the risk. Our son has no other options."

"I'm afraid my answer is still no."

The following day, Marianne leaves another message detailing the reasons John is the perfect candidate for stem cells. "Except for the SMA, he's very healthy."

Her next message is blunt. "We will lose him without you."

By week's end, after a dozen pleas, the doctor agrees. "You must get him here on time. Stem cells are matched by specific criteria that are unique for him."

A few days later, the entire family takes a road trip to Atlanta. Vera comes along to watch the children while John receives stem cells. Robert will meet them at the clinic. As soon as they settle into their hotel rooms, Vera tells them to get going.

"Thanks, Ma. We couldn't do this without you."

At the clinic, an oversized room partitioned with privacy screens, Marianne counts fifteen other patients and their families. Nurses and doctors walk around, talking with patients on stretchers or in wheelchairs along with the lucky few who can walk. Marianne feels connected to these men and women, each one fighting for life.

"This place looks nothing like a hospital," Robert says. "I hope you don't expect a miracle."

"That's exactly what John needs," she says.

"Medicine doesn't work that way. Science either."

"I'm certain we made the right decision." She is not the least bit afraid.

To start the transfusion of stem cells, the nurse looks for a vein in John's arms. When she doesn't find a good one, the doctor tries. He wraps a rubber band around John's upper arm and taps.

"Your son has no usable vein," the doctor says. "He needs a PICC line and a port for the infusion. You need to take him to the emergency room across town. I'll send a nurse with you. You have to hurry."

Rick speeds down unlit roads as the nurse shouts directions from the back seat.

"Slow down," Marianne screams.

"There's no time for that," Rick says.

At the hospital, the doctor looks at John. "I don't think I can help him."

"You have to," Marianne says. "He's supposed to get stem cells today."

"I can't guarantee anything." When the doctor approaches later, his face ashen and his tie unfastened, Marianne thinks the worst has happened.

"Oh no. John is gone."

"Not so," the doctor tells them. "It was tricky but we were able to put in a PICC line. He's ready for the infusion."

They arrive back at the clinic with minutes to spare. The doctor waves them forward. Before the infusion begins, Marianne leans in.

"I understand you're a Rabbi and a doctor. Can we start with a prayer?" The doctor closes his eyes and speaks in a soft voice. She feels the power of his words and trusts that John is in good hands.

During the infusion, a man nearby begins to sing. Others join in until it seems that everyone in the room is singing for the sun to come out tomorrow, no matter what happens today. The moment is tender and sad, and Marianne is overcome with affection for these strangers.

The doctor discharges John after three days of infusions. At the hotel, they pack up for the drive home.

"What is that smell?" Vera holds her nose.

"The doctor told us John would smell like bad oysters for a few days," Marianne says.

"A few days? I'm not sure I can take it that long."

Rick grabs a suitcase. "I'll be outside."

Amber rushes out with him, holding Robby's hand. "We'll wait in the car."

Only Britney is immune. "I don't smell anything." She bounces from bed to bed.

All of a sudden, John begins to choke on something lodged in his throat. Marianne stands paralyzed, too stunned to move. Vera grabs the baby and flips him over on her lap. She cups her hand, and pounds John's back like she's beating a drum. She moves her hand up and down his back until he spits up enough phlegm and is able to breathe.

"You saved him, Ma. I can't believe what you did."

"You would have done the same thing."

"I didn't know what to do, but you did. You saved his life."

It's a helpless feeling, not knowing what to do for your child. (Marianne)

We were brought up that you turn your baby and pat him on his back. So, when John was choking, I turned him over and patted his back. It was a natural thing. After we made it home, they brought him to the hospital to see about his breathing and that's when it all started. (Vera)

Vera is one of the most perceptive people I know. I'd put her up against any doctor with her ability to know when something is wrong and what to do. (Rick)

SIX TO SEVEN MONTHS OLD

TAKE A STAND

Once they are back home, they schedule John with a pediatric pulmonologist hoping to learn how to help their son's breathing. The morning of his appointment, John is quieter than usual. His chest hardly rises with each breath. His skin's tinted gray. At the office, the nurse says the doctor is running late. Rick thumbs through a magazine while Marianne holds John. After an hour, the doctor arrives.

"Let's have a look at your son," he says.

John seems to stop breathing as soon as he is put in the doctor's hands. "Call for a cart," the doctor yells out. "We have to intubate. It's the only way." They sign documents the nurse puts before them as John is wheeled away.

"Do you know what 'intubation' is?" Marianne asks Rick.

"I don't, but he said it's the only way."

Hours later when they are finally able to see John, he has a tube between his lips that goes down his throat. The other end is connected to a machine.

"The ventilator is breathing for him," the doctor says. "His lungs are shot. One collapsed. The other is too weak to support the whole body."

"When can he go home?" Marianne says.

"His lungs need to work properly for him to go home. At this point, it's too early to know when."

Marianne calls home right away. "The doctors want to keep your brother overnight," she tells the twins. "Is it okay if Rick and I stay at the hospital? Grandma can watch you."

"Why wouldn't it be alright," they say. "John needs you."

John sleeps under a labyrinth of hoses, his face crisscrossed with medical tape. Doctors disagree on the best way to care for him. One resident turns John on his left side for better breathing; another lays John on the right side. They disagree about ventilator settings and oxygen saturation.

"Do you think they're guessing?" Marianne says.

"Isn't this supposed to be a good hospital?" Rick says.

"Maybe John is their first SMA patient? Oh my God. Maybe he's the first one they've seen. What are we going to do?"

In the morning, the doctor admits John for further tests. "He still can't go home. His lungs are no better."

"How long will that take?" Marianne says. "We have other children at home to care for."

"I wish I knew. When we removed the breathing tube earlier today, he took a few breaths, but we had to intubate again in less than a minute. He has to be able to breathe on his own." After the doctor leaves, they watch John sleep.

"We both can't stay," Marianne says.

"You're right. All our kids need stability."

"I'll stay with John." There's no doubt in her mind.

"You sure?"

"Are you sure? You'll have the rest of it -- the twins, Robby, the house, your job." She smiles. "My mother."

"I'll come by after I drop the girls at school."

"Bring me an Everything Bagel and regular coffee?"

He nods. "I'll come by again after work. Veggie Burger and Diet Coke for dinner?"

"Sounds like a plan," she says.

Marianne marks the beginning of each day with the food he brings. Beyond that, it becomes difficult to track time. She does not leave John's bedside except to use the bathroom. When she steps away, she talks through the open door.

"Mommy's here, John."

She can't bear the thought that he might consider himself all alone in this hospital room. When the nurses push her out during shift changes, she sinks into an oversized chair and holds her head in her hands. Little by little her world narrows to this place, this room, this minute. She grieves that she cannot hold her son. She talks to him non-stop. She prays to the God of her understanding, the one who wants the best for all her children.

Many days she is angry. Angry that it takes so long to get the doctors' attention, angry that they have no answers; sometimes she is so angry she wants to throw up. She doesn't dare cry because she is certain the tears would never stop. She is so afraid of losing him she can barely breathe, yet she refuses to give up hope. Her desire to believe in his survival pushes aside the intense fear.

Rick brings the girls and Robby to visit on weekends. The children fawn over John and say they are fine. They assure her that school is good, Grandma takes care of them, and people bring food every day.

"I miss you so much," Marianne says.

Robert comes to the hospital after work. With his tie loosened, her brother sits at John's bedside reading the Daily News sports pages to his nephew.

"How much longer," Marianne asks the doctor.

"His condition still has not improved."

"Let us take him home anyway. He can get better there, with his brother and sisters." Her voice carries the pain and anguish of missing them.

"You don't understand," the doctor says. "He cannot breathe without the ventilator. The last time we removed the breathing tube, he lasted on his own only a few seconds before we had to intubate again. He's not getting better."

"I don't know what to do," Marianne says to Karen when she stops by for a visit.

"Don't be afraid," Karen says. "Doctors make decisions about patients based on what they see. There is so much more to John than what is visible to the eye."

Marianne points to the breathing tube. "What about that?"

"Look at that boy," Karen says. "There's no doubt that John is in charge of his life."

Later that night, one of the resident doctors adjusts John's ventilator settings.

"He looks weak, doesn't he?" Marianne says.

"When he first came in, none of us thought he would make it," the resident says.

"He received stem cells. Did that help?"

"Maybe that's why he's alive."

He's alive. The words startle her. She's so worried about losing him, she forgets he's here right now.

The next day, the nurses urge her to leave the hospital for a little while. "The sun is out," they say. "You should take a walk. Go home for some rest."

"I'm not leaving without him," Marianne says.

"We don't know when that will be. At the very least get some fresh air."

"I know you mean well, but we came in together and we will leave together." She stands by his bedside, wondering what he thinks of all this.

"You passed the six-month deadline, John, as few others have. What happens now? Do you want us to fight for you?"

His eyes, clear and bright, talk to her.

"I'll take that as yes."

Later that night, Marianne runs it by Rick. "I hope I'm reading him right."

"That kid had plenty of opportunities to crap out," Rick says. "He wants a chance."

Early one morning, John's doctor approaches her. "We need to talk."

"My husband is on his way," Marianne says. "We have to wait for him." After morning rounds, the doctor looks for them.

"Extubating is not easy. Many things can go wrong when we remove the tube. We will try again but if he cannot breathe without assistance, we want your permission to let him go."

Let him go? Marianne remembers when a veterinarian used those words for the family cat, but never imagined a doctor would want that for their child.

"We don't agree with that," Rick says.

Thank God he's reading my mind.

"Your son has no options. There's nothing we can do."

"We want you to keep trying," Rick says.

"Then what? What's your plan B?"

"My wife and I will figure something out." After the doctor leaves, Marianne calls her brother.

"I wish I had something to offer," Robert says. "All the

doctors I spoke with said the same thing."

"We need a family meeting," she tells Rick.

"Tomorrow after school," he says. "I'll bring the kids."

The next day, the twins kiss her cheek when they arrive, while Robby wraps his arms around her neck. Marianne treasures their affections, and nuzzles them all with kisses. "I'm sorry I missed your track meet," she says.

"Our team's not so good this year," Britney says.

"What? I love to watch you run. I miss that."

"John is attached to more machines than I knew existed," Amber says. "Is he going to die?"

"The doctors say he's not getting any better." With a calm voice, she delivers the hard information. "They say there is nothing more they can do, and they want us to let him go."

"We can't give up on John," Amber says.

Britney agrees.

Before the extubation procedure, the doctor stops in John's room where Marianne and Karen sit by his bedside. "Don't get your hopes up."

"Maybe the doctors are right," Marianne tells Karen.

"Don't get caught up in appearances. Instead of worrying,

focus on the end result you want. If you remember that miracles can happen, you can create a different reality from what the doctors say is possible."

Marianne wants John to know he has a choice. "If this is too much for you, go to the Blessed Mother Mary, and Mommy will be there as soon as she can." She puts her face close to his. "Or if you want to, you can live with your family who loves you very much and Mommy will try hard to help you." She kisses his face. "Do what you need to do."

In the waiting room, the women hang on to each other. Robert sits in a corner chair, shading his eyes. Rick paces the hall. Later, the doctor tells them that John survived the procedure.

"Halleluiah," they sing.

"Don't get too excited," the doctor says. "He's not out of the woods by a long shot. Marianne turns away from the doctor's list of complications and runs to John's room. He's connected to the ventilator with a tube down his throat, but his eyes greet her with a smile. She sighs at the sight of him.

"You are a brave boy." He stares at her face. "You made your decision, John, and Mommy will keep her promise." *I wish I knew where to start.*

The doctors told my mom and stepdad that their best option was to let my brother go. My family went back and forth discussing what should be done. We all came to the same conclusion. Life is too precious to throw away. Each life is worth fighting for. My brother stayed in the hospital for three months. Every day my mom told us that John might not live through the night and to prepare for the worst. I was unsure what the future held for John and my family. (Amber, seventh-grade essay)

I like to stay close to the house because there is always something happening with John. (Britney)

EIGHT TO NINE MONTHS OLD

BRAVE NEW LIFE

Her friend Jeannie stops by the hospital to see John. "I'm sorry it's been so long."

"You saw him after he was born," Marianne says.

"That was a few months ago. Time is funny. Can you believe it's been a year and a half since 9-11? Rod and I still go to memorial services every week."

"I've lost all sense of time in this place."

"How is John?"

"The doctors are not optimistic."

"Did I ever tell you about my husband's friend from the

firehouse? That's why I came. Rod keeps asking if I talked to you about Manny."

"I don't remember that name."

"After Rod's firehouse collapsed in 9-11, he transferred to Manny's station in the Bronx. He has a seven-year-old son with the same disease as John."

"That's not possible," Marianne says, confused. "Children with SMA1 don't live past age two."

"I'm almost a hundred percent sure. Rod and I saw him at last year's Christmas party. He uses a wheelchair."

Rick dismisses the story when Marianne tells his him. "One of the doctors would have said something."

"What if they didn't know?"

"How could they not know? Aren't they experts?"

Manny visits the hospital a few nights later. "I hope you don't mind. I heard so much about your son, I had to see for myself." He pulls a small photograph from his pocket. "My son has the same disease."

The next night, Manny brings more pictures. "This is one of the machines we use. Because of SMA, my son isn't able to cough, so this does it for him. It's called a cough assist. He hands Marianne a piece of paper. "You can have the machine delivered here."

"How do you know so much?"

"We learned from Dr. John Bach. He works at a hospital in Newark, New Jersey."

"This is the first we're hearing about him," Rick says.

"We didn't know about him either," Manny says. "We met another couple whose child has this disease; they told us."

The next day, Rick leaves a message for Dr. Bach while Marianne orders a cough assist machine. When it arrives during Manny's next visit, the doctor blocks delivery to John's room.

"That machine is not part of his treatment plan." While the doctor stands his ground, Marianne feels a pang of how much she misses her other children. They have all given up a lot to help John and now, when something possibly could help, the doctor disagrees. Anger surges through her center.

"My husband and I agree on this." Her voice is strong, confident and unwavering.

"You will have to sign a disclaimer," the doctor says.

"Whatever you need."

Manny places the cough assist mask on John's face, covering his nose and mouth. "You can learn to do this."

The next day, a new doctor visits John. "I heard about your son." Marianne has a bad feeling about this. "I know what happens to babies with SMA1," the doctor says.

"You don't know John."

"When your son is fifteen, he will hate you for making him live like this." After the doctor leaves, Marianne savors the image of John as an angry teenager.

"When you are fifteen," she tells him, "you can hate me all you want."

Once John is more stable and after the discharge papers are signed, a private ambulance, outfitted with a ventilator and other emergency equipment, transports John to the New Jersey hospital while Marianne and Rick follow in their car. Dr. Bach meets them at the Emergency Room entrance.

"Why did you wait this long to bring him?" A deep frown creases his forehead. "Your son is very sick, maybe the sickest I've seen, but we will do our best. We will start respiratory treatments right away."

They sit for hours waiting until Dr. Bach brings them to the recovery room. "We were able to successfully remove the breathing tube. He now uses nose prongs. We call it noninvasive ventilation or NIV. They are connected to a Bi-Pap, which has different settings than a ventilator."

"What happens next?" Rick says.

"Your son needs to recover from what he's been through.

In the meantime, twice a day, he'll receive respiratory treatments to improve his breathing."

"What are his chances?"

"We will use the cough assist to loosen secretions, then the suction machine to vacuum them out. With a little luck, your son can make it."

In a few days, John looks healthier. His skin is bright for the first time in months. He gains a few ounces of weight. He's awake more than asleep. One morning, Dr. Bach hands Marianne the cough assist mask. "It's time for you to try."

"I'm not ready."

"Other parents have learned. Once you learn, your son can go home."

"Home?" She is surprised to hear the word.

"It will be touch and go for a while, but if he gets through the first few years, he can have a life."

"What about the quality of his life?" Rick asks.

"Quality of life is subjective." Dr. Bach pulls a small photo from his pocket. "If you knew I taught classes, worked with families like yours, wrote articles and books, and didn't have a spare minute to myself, you might not think much about the quality of my life. The thing is, I love my life." He hands Rick the sonogram image.

"I'm about to become a father. Twins."

"What about the impact on families?" Rick says.

"The one common element is love. There is so much love in each family."

Marianne holds the mask on John's face. She counts in her head to steady her hands. After the cough assist, she tries to slide the red suction tube down his throat when her gag reflex kicks in.

"I can't do it."

"He doesn't have the same reflex as you do," Dr. Bach says. "He doesn't feel it like you would."

"What if I mess up?"

"Try not to. As you get to know him, you will learn more. For now, take it one treatment at a time. "

She slips the silicone tube between his lips and pushes, careful not to overjudge the space. Afterwards, she sits on her hands to hide their tremor.

For ten more days, John remains at the hospital in Newark, where he receives respiratory treatments twice a day, along with other medical care. The staff trains Marianne and Rick to use the cough assist and the suction machine. They demonstrate how an Ambu-Bag works. They explain why oxygen saturation matters. When John is discharged, Marianne worries that it's too soon.

"I wouldn't let him go home if I didn't think you could take care of him," Dr. Bach says.

"I hope you're right."

"Don't be afraid to dial 9-1-1."

Vera waits at the front door with Robby. She touches her daughter's shoulder as Marianne enters the house. "You don't look so good," Vera says.

"That's an understatement, Ma." Her pants hang loose on her hips, she hasn't worn make-up in three months, and her hair needs to be washed. *I'm a shadow of my former self.*

"Mom!" The twins draw out the word into three syllables. "When did you get home?" The dogs are there, too, pushing into Marianne and howling. They sit together, resuscitating themselves with each other. Later, she drags them all into John's room where stuffed animals have been replaced with the Bi-Pap, the cough assist, and an assortment of medical tubes, hoses and bandages. She tries to remember the purpose of each item.

There's no way I can do this.

Vera cooks supper the way she did on Sundays when Marianne was growing up. Pasta, meatballs, sausages, and crusty Italian bread. Marianne sits at the table with both boys in her lap.

"Hurry up, Ma. We're hungry."

Vera fills a bowl for her daughter. "Have a taste."

"Oh my God, Ma." Marianne wipes her mouth. "I never tasted food this good." She eats until she is stuffed.

Later that night, Rick reads off the numbers on the oximeter. "Do you remember what they mean?"

"I hope so," she says. They don't move from John's bedside until he opens his eyes in the morning. When he does, they are amazed to see that he made it through the first night with them.

"We did something right," Rick says.

"Let's hope we remember what it is."

"Maybe we won't need 9-1-1," Rick says.

"We'll need it. It's just a question of when."

The next day she carries the phone with 9-1-1 on speed dial. The baby's life depends on a respiratory treatment done properly twice a day. She is terrified of making a mistake.

They sit and watch him sleep. They check his feeding tube to be sure it's unclogged. They check the settings on the Bi-Pap. They check his oxygen numbers. They watch his chest to be sure it rises and falls. They repeat the checks throughout the night, taking turns, monitoring each other as well as the machines.

"I'm impressed how much we seem to know," Rick says.

"Whatever we're doing is working because he's alive."

The first time John struggles to breathe, Marianne puts the Ambu-Bag mask on his face and squeezes, forcing in air. When that doesn't work, she calls 9-1-1 and the EMTs revive John.

A few days after John is home, Rashida knocks at the front door. "I tried to get in touch," she tells Marianne. "No one could tell me what happened."

"I'm sorry I didn't call," Marianne says. "It was crazy." The women stand at John's bedside. "He is much weaker than when you first saw him. Is there anything you can do?"

Rashida touches John's shoulder. "Are you ready to get to work John?"

He smiles.

"Wait until you find out what work means," Rashida says. "We are going to get along." She gently stretches John's legs; first one, then the other. She massages his feet. "Little by little John will get stronger."

Rashida's words lift Marianne's spirit. Each night, they experiment on what works for John and what doesn't work. Little by little, through trial and error, he does get stronger. His arms and legs are more flexible. His breathing seems more stable.

During the waning days of summer, the sun feels warmer than ever before. The sky is a deeper shade of blue. The twins are happier. Rick moves easier. Robby doesn't leave his mother's side. Marianne holds the boys, watches her daughters, talks with Rick, and drinks coffee with Vera.

Every night since they brought John home from the hospital, Marianne cooks dinner from ingredients she finds in the pantry and refrigerator. She chops vegetables, broils chicken, or boils spaghetti. Each night, the family sits together. Many evenings, John sleeps through the entire meal. Other times his eyes are open for the first few minutes or wakes up at the very end. Usually, they are hungry though some nights no one seems to have an appetite.

During dinner, the twins talk about school, friends, teachers, and grades. No matter what is going on with John's breathing or his medical condition, dinner time is when the other children talk about themselves. Sometimes there's not a lot to say; other times the girls talk into the night. They try to keep the talk upbeat. Some nights, they sit together long after they've finished eating; other nights, they can't wait to get back to their separate lives. Putting together a meal for the family helps Marianne navigate the uncertainty of each day. The nightly routine seems to help the others, too. Together, they help each other through this new reality.

Dr. Bach insisted that the parents know best. I always respected him for this. (Rick)

Things changed when we found Dr. Bach. Before that, it was all about how and when we were going to lose our child. John was eight months old when the whole thing changed to a situation where John is fragile, but with a cough assist and respiratory treatment, he can breathe with a Bi-Pap and maybe without a Bi-Pap, and he can live his life. I was blown away by the change. Dr. Bach said, 'Give him a few years to grow, then he can help himself.' So that became the goal. (Marianne)

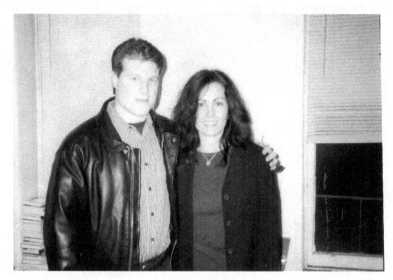

Marianne and Rick, 2000

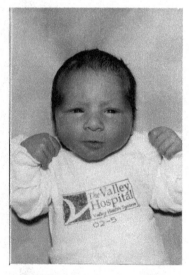

John at birth, August 8, 2002

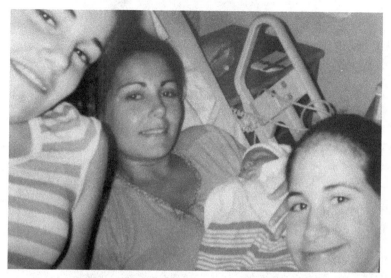

Twins, Amber and Britney, with newborn John, 2002

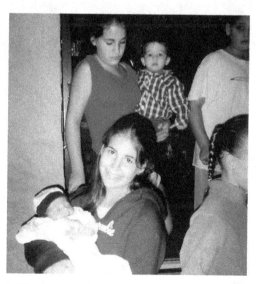

Amber, Robby, Britney, and John at Labor Day Barbeque, September 1, 2002

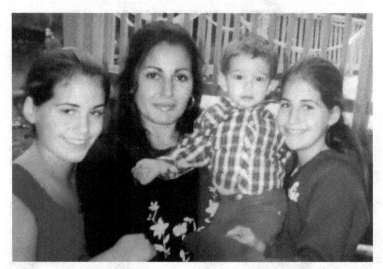

Amber, Britney, Robby with Marianne at Labor Day Barbeque, September 1, 2002

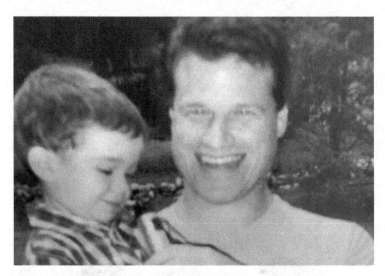

Rick with Robby at Labor Day Barbeque, September 1, 2002

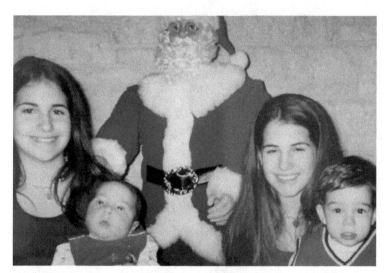

John's first Christmas, December 2002

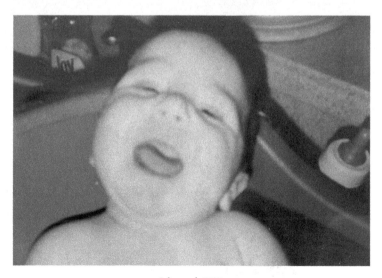

John, early 2003

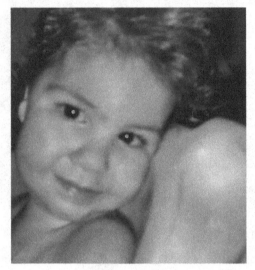

John,2003

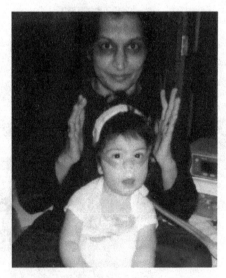

John with Rashida,2004

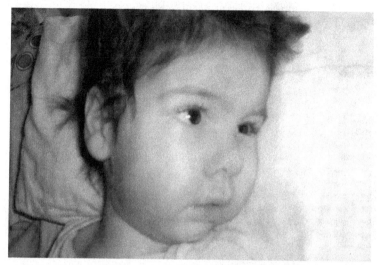

John,2003

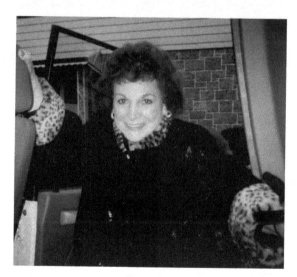

Vera,2007

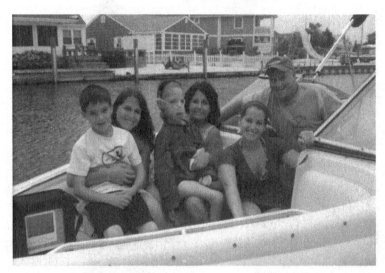

John, with his parents, Robby, Amber and Britney, at the Jersey shore, Summer 2008

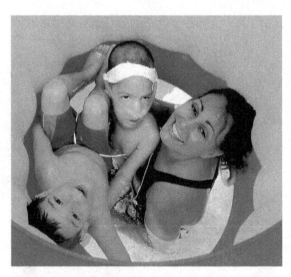

John, with Robby and Marianne, backyard pool, Summer 2008

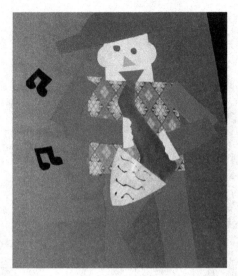

John's artwork, 2014

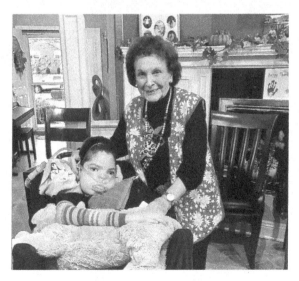

John with his grandmother, Vera, 2016

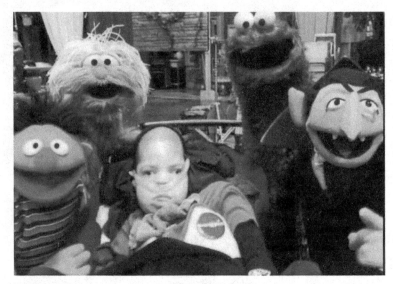

John visiting the Sesame Street Studio, Queens, NY, 2016

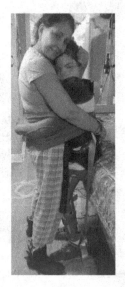

John standing with his mom, 2017

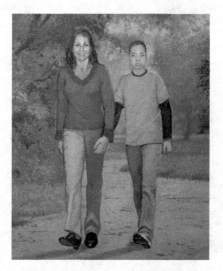

Painting commissioned by Amber, Britney and Robby for their Mom's Christmas gift, 2016

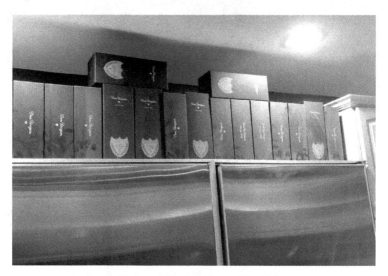

Years of champagne bottles celebrating John's life, 2018

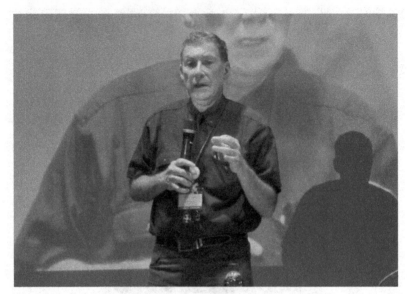

Dr. John Bach

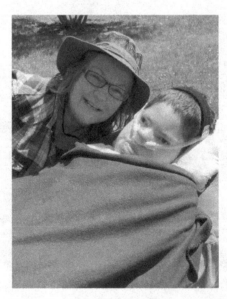

John with author, 2018

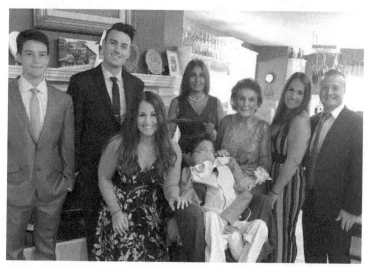

John attending family wedding with Marianne, Vera, Robby (left), and Amber (left) and Britney (right) with their boyfriends, 2019

TEN MONTHS TO TWO YEARS OLD

HOW SWEET IT IS

In the early days of caring for John, everyone tiptoes around. He is so fragile, it's hard enough to keep him alive from one minute to the next. Everyone does their best, but the diagnosis is a game-changer, no doubt about that.

The girls are grieving their father's death and now face the possible loss of their brother. Rick seems lost. Marianne tries to be available for everyone, but with a child this sick, she has to be prepared that John's condition can change any minute. She is nervous when not next to John's bed where she can keep an eye on him. Robby, a toddler, takes it all in stride.

When people ask how she's doing, she says she is fine.

They give John statues -- St. Jude, Sacred Heart of Jesus, and Mary, the Holy Mother of God. Others offer peace flags or essential oils. The saints share space on the altar above John's bed. The flags hang along the bed's railing. As a nightly ritual, she massages John's feet with frankincense oil.

Their first summer home, when John is not quite one year old, is filled with the pain of knowing they could lose him. At the same time, he brings joy into their lives; John's personality has begun to take form and he is fun to be around. Rick decorates the backyard with plastic palm trees and party lights. He cleans out the pool. The girls invite friends for burgers and hot dogs. Everyone pretends they're on vacation.

Marianne functions better when she believes things are happening as they are supposed to happen. Yet, despite her efforts to see the best, thoughts of SMA torment her. She can't help comparing John to other kids his age who don't have the disease. If John didn't have the disease, he'd crawl and might take his first steps. He would sit without help; scribble with crayons. These are the things their other children did when they were John's age. She mourns for what he cannot do.

"Why did this happen to John?" she asks Robert one night.

"Nothing happened to John." Robert's response is quick.

"SMA is a part of who he is. It's how he was born."

"I'd give anything for him not to have it."

"Then he wouldn't be the child you call your son."

"What?"

"Do you know what I mean?" he says.

She promises to think about it.

"Is it fair?" Vera asks her daughter the next day.

"Is what fair, Ma?"

"If John ends up in a wheelchair, is it fair to make him live like that?"

"John wants us to fight for him. He wants to live." She wishes her mother didn't need an explanation.

That night, John stares at her during his bath. "Boo-boo," he says. "Boo-boo."

"Yes, John, you have a boo-boo called SMA. Don't worry. Mommy will help fix your boo-boo."

To celebrate his first birthday, Marianne bakes a cake with the girls and wraps presents. Rick helps Robby hang balloons.

"Happy Birthday," they sing. "You did it, John."

"Yay, John." The girls shout like cheerleaders.

She can't believe how fast they grew up. They'll start high

school in a month and soon will be teenagers. Then, they'll want to spend summer weekends at the Jersey Shore with girlfriends. She'll say no, of course, but they'll go anyway as she did.

"Keep an eye on them," she tells Rick one morning.

"We're only going to school."

She laughs. "You know what I mean."

John's second Christmas is better than his first when the doctors gave him less than two months to live. This New Year's Eve, Rick stashes another champagne bottle on top of the refrigerator. A few weeks later, Robby wakes up with a runny nose and a cough. Marianne isolates him from the others. She wears a face mask and gloves when she cares for him, then scrubs herself clean and changes clothes when she leaves Robby's bedside. Despite all the safety precautions, John catches a cold, too.

His secretions build up fast and his oxygen level drops. Marianne gives him additional respiratory treatments that do little to stop the build-up of secretions in his airways. The next day, she suctions him every two hours and the pediatrician sends a nurse with antibiotics, but John's condition does not improve.

"He sounds junky," Marianne says. "I don't think we can wait any longer."

When the EMTs arrive, they load John into the ambulance.

"You have to take him to Dr. Bach," she tells them.

"Your son is too sick to go that far."

"Can you go with them to the hospital?" she asks Rick. "I promised Robby I'd stay here until he's better."

"I'll call from the hospital," Rick says.

As the ambulance speeds away flashing lights and blasting sirens, the twins tug at her. "We have a spelling test tomorrow. Can you quiz us?"

Marianne isn't sure what to do. Should she talk with them about what happened with John, or follow their lead? "Who's got the spelling list?" she says. They run through the words twice.

When she arrives at the hospital the next day, she isn't prepared for how frail John looks.

"Your son has RSV," the doctor says. "It stands for Respiratory Syncytial Virus. I'm not going to lie. Your son might not make it."

She doesn't want to hear this. "Please, doctor. He's only been back with us a short time."

Rick telephones Dr. Bach for advice.

"Bring him to me as soon as you can."

When John is stable enough to be moved while intubated and breathing with a ventilator, he is transferred by ambulance to the Newark NJ hospital. Marianne feels a sense of relief. *If he is going to get better, it will happen there.*

Hours after Dr. Bach admits John to the pediatric intensive care unit, he brings them an update on his condition. "After a few unsuccessful attempts, we extubated and replaced the breathing tube with nasal prongs. He is now on noninvasive ventilation with the Bi-Pap."

Marianne stays with John in his hospital room, while Rick heads north to the house. The first days are rough for John, but he gets through them and after a week he looks stronger and his eyes are brighter.

"He can go home soon," Dr. Bach says. "But his lungs are weaker now, so he'll also need the Bi-Pap for when he sleeps."

A few days after John's discharge, Marianne realizes he hasn't said a word since the RSV intubation. No gurgles or sounds. *It's unfair.* She wants to scream. How can he tell her he needs help? How will she know what he wants? Full of despair and uncertainty, she calls Dr. Bach.

"I can't imagine that life for him," she says.

"I know many people who carry on after a change like this. You can too."

Marianne isn't so sure. All she can do it seems is put one

foot in front of the other.

"Snap out of it," Vera says. "Whatever is going on, you have to snap out of it."

"Nothing's going on, Ma."

"Please. You walk around with that face."

"What face?"

"You know what I'm talking about. Your children are watching you. They need you. You have to take care of them all."

"I don't know if I can."

"You are stronger than you know."

Rashida visits the next day.

"Starting over may be too much for him," Marianne says.

"He's not starting over. He's starting from where he was. He knows much more than when we first worked with him. We will start slow and see how it goes."

"Look at him," Marianne says.

"He made progress before," Rashida says.

"Maybe he's gone as far as he can."

"He will show us what he can do."

Marianne gently touches John's face. "I'll do anything to help him."

That night, she considers her own words. Is she willing to

do anything? If so, then she needs to forgive herself for carrying this disease to John. She also needs to forgive the doctor who kept the diagnosis from them and the ones who urged them to let their baby go. If she doesn't forgive it all, the grudge will choke her.

Rashida works with John at night, on days off and on weekends. She's there so often, Robby calls her his "aunt." The twins tell friends Rashida is family though they aren't sure which side; they often sit with her while she exercises John. Rick clears out a room for her to have private space. One day, Marianne gives Rashida a photo of John.

"Will you pray for him?"

"I pray for John every day," Rashida says. "I pray for your family as much as I pray for my own. I will put his picture on my altar." She pulls a small square from her bag. "Perhaps you want to add this to John's altar. It's an image of Aqa Maula, the spiritual leader of the Muslim sect I belong to." Marianne puts the image next to John's sacred crystals and the Holy Water.

"It looks good up there. Thank you."

"I hope Aqa Maula gives you the same comfort I find in my devotion and deep love for the Mother Mary you pray to."

Marianne suspects that when she looks back, she will see that Rashida was an angel who stepped into their world and changed them all.

No matter how many calm medical days John has in a row, Marianne keeps 9-1-1 on speed dial. One night, when the electricity cuts off without notice, the entire street goes dark.

"We should have a generator," Rick says.

"How did we not plan for this?" She calls 9-1-1 and tries not to panic. All she has to do is keep him breathing until the paramedics arrive.

Without considering whether her idea will work, she pulls the end of the breathing tube out of the Bi-Pap and leaves the other end connected to the nasal prongs. She blows into the tube until his chest rises with air. When the air leaves his lungs, she blows into his breathing tube a second time. With each rise and fall of his chest, she knows he is getting enough air to stay alive. She continues blowing her breath into his breathing tube for twenty-five minutes until the ambulance arrives.

The EMT pulls an extension cord into John's room. "We set up a generator outside." He plugs in the Bi-Pap and reconnects the breathing tube. "How's it going?"

"John's fine, but I'm a little winded." After the EMT leaves, Robby shuffles in. "How's my big boy?" Almost four years old, Robby is fair-haired like his dad. "Do you know how special you are? Did you know there's a special song for you?"

Marianne kicks her legs like a Rockette. "Let's do the Robby dance." She puts a tune to the words, and sings. "The Robby dance. Let's do the Robby dance." She twirls him around the room. "We're having fun doing the Robby dance."

On John's second birthday, Marianne wants to celebrate his most amazing feat, something few others have accomplished. The doctors said it wasn't possible, but he proved them wrong. *You beat the odds, John. My uncles should take you to Vegas. You'd win them a fortune.* Though she's grateful for the two years, she wants more. Everyone wants more time with John. They adapted their lives to his and they are happy.

They throw John a birthday party that's as fancy as a wedding. Long buffet tables draped with white linen are lined with food trays: sausage and peppers; lasagna; deli meats; cheeses; and salads. Chicken and burgers are served up at two grilling stations. Coolers overflow with beer and soft drinks. Vera's brother mixes up Cosmopolitans. They invite everyone who knows John along with everyone else they could think of. One young neighbor shows off his new baby brother. "Is your brother a mover?" Robby asks. "Some babies move, but my brother doesn't."

As Marianne takes in the excitement, she wishes she invited the experts who saw no future for John. They were correct that he has SMA, but wrong about everything else. If they were here, she would show off John's straight spine, the way he holds up his head without help, and how he sits with cushions. Those doctors could not see beyond their diagnosis and prognosis. They could not see the possibility of life for John. If those doctors saw the love that surrounds this child, would they see a quality life? Would they understand why his parents tried so hard?

"Look at my grandson," Vera tells everyone within earshot. "Isn't John a beautiful boy?"

"Ma, I hope I have your energy when I'm eighty."

"I hope so, too."

On a makeshift stage, Robert tunes his guitar while a crowd gathers around. "How you all doing?" The crowd whoops and hollers. He taps the microphone. "Testing one, two, three." Robert's performance lasts well into the night, filling the summer air with tender melodies and sweet music. Marianne looks at the faces around her. No doubt about it: there is so much love and happiness that surrounds John.

Now I understand what my brother meant when he said John wouldn't be John if he didn't have SMA. Just like I was meant to have Amber, Britney, and Robby, I was meant to have John. And if John were any other way, he wouldn't be John. It was the smartest thing Robert ever said to me. I didn't understand it at the time though it would have helped if I had. (Marianne)

THREE TO SIX YEARS OLD

STRONGER EVERY DAY

In his third year, Marianne calls 9-1-1 not as often as before but with a regularity that forces her to question her competency. "After all this time, you'd think I'd have it figured out," she says after the EMTs stabilize John one day.

"I think we're doing good," Rick says. "John is stable. That's all we can ask for."

None of it is easy. It's tough enough with a blended family of four children, but when one of them has life and death needs, there's no time or energy for anything else.

John's physical development continues to be a primary focus of his day-to-day therapy, besides the respiratory treatments that are the regular beginning and ending points of his day.

"It's time he learned to stand," Marianne says one day.

"What do you have in mind?" Rashida asks.

They buy a bucket seat online like the ones found in children's playgrounds, and hang it from the ceiling. When John sits strapped in the seat, his feet touch the ground; his legs have to work hard to keep them there. Beads of sweat dot his forehead. After two minutes, she lifts him out.

"That's a good start, John." She kisses his cheek. "Ooh, I'm addicted to kissing you." She buries herself in his neck, kissing him again and again.

He sits in the bucket seat every day after that. Week after week, he adds another minute of endurance. John's body grows stronger with Rashida's physical therapy and his time in the bucket seat. After a month of daily sits, he lasts five minutes.

John took to the water right away as a baby and since then, has daily baths. When he outgrew the sink, he floated in the bathtub. Now, he uses a bigger indoor therapy pool every day for ninety minutes. The Bi-Pap stays dry on a shelf with an extra-long breathing tube connected to his nasal prongs. In the warm water, his arms and legs move with ease. As he sits on his mother's lap, she massages his spine to help it grow straight.

One doctor wants him to use a metal back brace. "With a solid brace to support his back, he can sit up unassisted for longer periods of time."

"Won't he collapse like wet noodles when the brace comes off?" Marianne says. "Isn't it better for him to strengthen his core muscles by using a soft brace?"

The doctor is unconvinced. "We recommend a hard brace for children like yours."

Children like mine? You don't know what he is capable of. She goes ahead with a soft brace for John. He uses it when watching television with his brother or sisters; with yoga blocks wedged against his sides and towels tucked under his neck, he sits with them on the couch.

John experiences a growth spurt when he turns four years old. His pediatrician says he's among the tallest of boys in his age group. The fall classes begin in the school district, and John becomes eligible for in-home occupational therapy. The school district sends Joan to assess him for services.

"Can you talk?" she asks him. "I bet you have a lot to say."

John stares at her.

"He talks in his own way," Marianne says.

"That's not good enough," Joan says. "He will have many

people in his life -- teachers, relatives and someday, his own friends. He has to talk with all of them."

"Watch me," she tells John. "Can you blink like this?" She opens and closes her eyes.

He imitates her blinking.

"Good. That's good. So, when you want to say yes, you blink your eyes twice." She blinks twice. "Okay, you try."

He follows her lead.

"Now when you want to say no, you roll your eyes like this." Her eyes make wide, bug-eyed circles.

John's left shoulder shakes with laughter.

"You try it."

He spins his eyes.

"He's smart," she tells Marianne. Three days a week Joan works with him, exercising his mouth and jaw against the weakening from SMA. One day she asks Marianne to sit with them. "He has something to show you." She looks at John. "Can you show your mother how you can say 'yes' with your voice?"

"Ah huh."

"Say it again."

"Ah huh."

"Beautiful," Marianne says.

Joan also teaches him to use a variety of adaptive equipment including a sling that holds his arm steady while another tool helps his hand grip things like a pencil or a paintbrush. One day, she attaches a spoon.

"Now you can help your mother make cookies."

Marianne takes out a bowl and blends the ingredients. "Your turn," she tells John. With his adaptive spoon and his arm in the sling, he mixes the batter with Joan's help.

"His grasp will improve as he gets older," she says.

As he gets older. Marianne never grows tired of hearing those words.

One day, Joan sets up a triangle of plastic bowling pins on the kitchen table. Marianne holds John in her lap while Robby sits by her side. Joan hands her the ball.

"Can you help John roll it into the pins?"

Marianne moves his arm backward then forward. She opens his hand to release the ball. It hits one pin before rolling off the table onto the floor.

"Good job," Joan says. "How about you, Robby? Do you want to try?" He takes the ball from John's hand, eyes the pins, and knocks them all down.

"Way to go, Robby." Marianne marvels at his easy

movement. She is happy for him, and at the same time overwhelmed with pain for John. He can't do what Robby can. What most kids can. That breaks her heart.

"I'm feeling sorry for myself," she tells Karen the next time they talk.

"How's that working for you?"

Marianne laughs. "It hasn't changed a thing."

"There's always hope."

"Only if I accept all my children as they are."

Rashida and Joan work together in a combined treatment they developed for John. They watch him closely as they move him; if he shows pain, they stop.

John outgrows the bucket seat as inches and pounds are added to his lean frame. A new device called a Stander is added to his routine. In the Stander, John is held upright and strapped in. Once again, the machine holds his body in place and his leg muscles burn with pain as he stands. He's bigger, so there's more weight for him to hold up. His first few times in the Stander, he barely lasts a minute. After a week of effort, he ekes out one more minute. After more than a month, he stands longer than five minutes.

Like any kid, though, John has lazy days when he does not want to work out. Marianne lets a day pass because she sometimes gives the other kids a pass on things they have to do, but she won't let John go beyond that. Without daily water therapy, his body tightens up, his muscles contract. If he misses too much physical therapy, his limbs move slower and are less flexible.

"You're training for the Olympics," Marianne says. "You have to train every day to keep in shape."

He rolls his eyes. No.

"Come on, John. Exercise strengthens your muscles. The Stander helps every part of your body. You have to."

He rolls his eyes again.

"You are as stubborn as the rest. Okay, how about this: five minutes in the Stander now gets you five more minutes of watching videos tonight?"

He blinks twice. When she lifts him out, his shirt is soaked through with sweat. The next day, with John in the Stander, Rashida and Joan put a small treadmill under his feet. With one on each side, they move his legs along the treadmill to give him a sense of how it feels to walk.

One warm afternoon, Robby speeds around the backyard on his tricycle. John's face beams with excitement.

"Do you want to try that?" Marianne says.

He blinks twice.

She feels his racing heart. "Okay, Mommy will figure something out." That night, she pulls out Robby's old tricycle. She adds a wide strap to each handlebar and a strap to each pedal. She duct tapes a tall board against the back.

"What do you think?" she asks Rick.

"It could work."

"He might get hurt," she says.

"We agreed we wouldn't hold our kids back, and that includes John."

"You're right. The truth is, I worry about Robby all the time, but don't stop him."

The next day, Marianne has John sit on the tricycle, his hands attached to the grip and his feet to the pedals. She straps him to the back board with extra-wide bandages. She secures his head in place with a bandana.

"Are you ready?"

He blinks twice.

She hunches over and pushes the tricycle to the end of the driveway. She picks up speed downhill.

"You're riding, John," she shouts. "This is how it feels to

ride a bike." She pushes him around the block twice more and then to the house. "Enough?"

He rolls his eyes.

"You want more?"

He blinks twice.

She laughs. "All my children want more."

The following year, the school district wants to add classes to John's home-based services where he will learn math, English and reading.

"He's busy," Marianne says. "Physical therapy, occupational therapy, respiratory therapy, and water therapy. He has no time to add anything else."

"All kids have busy days," the school rep says. "I bet your daughters have extracurricular activities, homework, and social calls from friends. Your son Robby probably has a schedule in pre-school. They all have to learn how to manage their days. John has to learn, too. He does not get a free pass when it comes to school."

The following week, his new teacher, Miss Laurie, meets him for the first time. She brings a box with holes on each end, and slides something into one of the holes.

"What's in the box, John?"

Marianne slides his hand through the other hole and helps him search for the hidden object.

"What is it?" Miss Laurie runs through a list of possibilities. "Is it a whistle? A piece of paper? A ball?"

He blinks twice. Marianne pulls out their hands.

"A ball. That's right."

"You're now part of the J-Team," Marianne tells Miss Laurie. "We all work together to help John. We will take our cues from him and work him as hard as he lets us."

One evening, Rick tells Marianne he wants to go out to dinner with her. "A few hours. It's our anniversary."

She can't imagine leaving John alone.

"We'll be five minutes away," Rick says. "And John has a nurse tonight."

At the restaurant, the waiter fills their water glasses and announces dinner specials. He brings them a basket of warm bread. Marianne looks around at the other diners and wonders whether any of them have a child with SMA. As they share appetizers, they try to make their time together as pleasant as possible. They talk about nothing in particular. The food is good. They are having a nice time. Marianne gets a call from the nurse before their main course arrives.

Rick motions for the waiter. "Can you pack the rest of our food to go?"

The same EMT shows up each time there's a call, and over time he's become friends with John. "Don't you think we love him as much as you do?" he asks Marianne.

One day, the EMT stops by between calls to say hello. During the unannounced visit, Britney frantically bursts through the front door.

"Where's John?" She bends over to catch her breath.

"With his teacher. What's wrong?"

"What do you mean, what's wrong? There's an ambulance out front."

"He stopped by to see your brother."

"Stopped by? Are you kidding? I thought something bad happened to John."

Amber walks in as the EMT is leaving. "What's wrong? What's going on?" she asks.

"He stopped by to visit John," Britney says. "With the ambulance. Can you believe it?"

"Aren't you're overreacting a little bit?" Marianne says.

"You always do this," Amber says.

"What do I do?"

"You think we shouldn't get upset over anything because we don't have problems like John's."

"You're right. John can't walk or talk or eat. He can't breathe. He can't move. Those are real problems."

"We have problems, too," Britney says. "Different ones."

That night Marianne tells her bother what happened with the girls. "Did I ruin them?"

"Go easy on yourself," Robert says. "We all ruin our kids at least a little. Every parent screws up."

She wishes she could pack it up like that, but she has to fix it if she can. One morning a few days later, she sits with the twins in the kitchen. "I'm here if you want to talk." At least she can tell them that. She hopes it's enough.

One night as she cooks dinner, John works out with the stationary bicycle that moves his legs as though he's peddling.

"You have to tell me how you feel." She talks to him from the kitchen in a loud voice. "Do you hear me? If something is wrong, you can say, 'Mama ow. Mama ow.' She's given this a lot of thought. "If you have an itch, you could say, 'Mama fly,' like a bug bit you. Do you understand?"

"Mama."

She runs to his room.

"That's it, John. If you need me, say my name." She adds another ten minutes to the exercise machine, then heads back to the kitchen to finish dinner.

"Mama ow."

She runs to his room, ready to fix whatever is wrong. When he sees her, his left shoulder moves up and down.

"Are you goofing on me?"

His shoulder bobs faster.

"That's enough, mister."

Back in the kitchen she hears him again.

"Mama."

I can't give in all the time. Then she worries it could be something serious, and she runs to his room.

And so, it goes. His voice restored, John calls out to his mother over and over that night, until she surrenders, sits by his bedside, and asks Rick to bring home take-out food.

After that, she teaches John more words. "Say, Robby." When John uses a particular sound for his brother's name, that becomes Robby's name. Marianne goes through the list: Amber, Britney, Robby, Dad, Grandma. Each name gets a unique sound.

As John gets more comfortable with the sound of his voice, he talks more, forming words with sounds, stringing them together to form sentences. In that way, he creates a language that she learns to understand. If she is unsure what he is saying, they walk through the alphabet together.

"What does the word start with, John? A? B? Does it start with C?" If he rolls his eyes, she continues, until the first letter is reached. "T? It starts with a T? Okay. What's the second letter. A? B?" She runs through the alphabet like that until he forms a complete thought.

One day, during an in-school visit with the administrator, Marianne meets a new speech therapist.

"Do you work with children at home?" Marianne asks.

"Yes, I do," Stephanie says. "And I have time in my schedule for another one." At their first meeting, they bond like old pals. She understands what John says, and he complies with her instructions.

"Direct your eyes to that button," she says. "We call it a cell. Once you do that, the whole word comes up so you don't have to go letter-to-letter with your eyes." In a short time, John learns how to move his eyes on a computer screen in order to tap enough cells to asks questions.

"I can't believe how fast he learns," Stephanie says. "He's learning to use up to thirty cells on multiple pages. Next, I'll show him how to use the Internet. Maybe we can get him a pen pal so he can send emails."

One day, Stephanie invites Marianne to sit in on John's classroom time. "He wants to show you something."

John focuses on the computer screen and open groups of cells. "How was your day?" the computer's voice says.

"How was my day?" Marianne says. "It was good."

"What did you do today?"

"I got to be your mother for another day. That made it a great day."

Watching him work on the computer, Marianne thinks he might be cross-eyed. She explains to the ophthalmologist how John seems to look in two directions at the same time. After examining John's vision, the doctor confirms Marianne's suspicions.

"It's remarkable, really," the eye doctor says. "To accommodate for his limited mobility, he's learned to separate his fields of vision so his eyes can work independently and take in more. He'll need glasses when he starts walking."

When he starts walking. She's amazed by how very normal that sounds.

As he learns to operate the computer with more ease, the J-Team connects it to the television so John can turn it on himself.

One night, while his mother watches TV with him, John secretly turns it off. Marianne switches it on with the remote, but John switches it off again.

"Rick," she calls out. "We need a new TV."

He stands at the doorway, holding a sandwich. What's wrong with this one?"

"I don't know. It keeps turning off." Out of the corner of her eye, she sees John's left shoulder jump. She pretends to gasp. "John Donato Del Guercio." She tries to sound stern. "Did you do that?" His shoulder moves faster. "Rick." She draws out his name like a child. "John's messing with me."

John laughs so hard, he almost gags on secretions, which makes him laugh harder. Marianne slips the red tube between his lips, slides it down his throat, and turns on the suction machine.

"You are hilarious, John."

He goofs on Robby, too. One autumn day, the boys pick apples at a farm in New York State. Marianne pushes John in a wagon, while Robby walks alongside. When a car veers towards them, she yanks the cart out of the way, tossing John in a pile of leaves. Robby runs to John with Marianne close behind. On the ground, they both brush the leaves off John.

"You are a good big brother."

"Is he laughing?" Robby says.

They watch John's shoulder bounce.

Soon, John outgrows the stroller he's used for years but is not yet strong enough for a wheelchair. He needs another way to be mobile enough for outdoor activities. Otherwise, he will stay camped out in his room. With the right contraption and the portable Bi-Pap, Marianne would be able to take him for walks around the neighborhood.

One day, after walking around a hardware store looking for ideas, she buys a three-foot-high utility cart that can hold a hundred pounds, more weight than John and the Bi-Pap combined. The Bi-Pap fits on a side-shelf with room for emergency medical supplies. With a mattress on top and straps to secure him, John now has a mobile bed.

The first time she lays him on the bed, his body trembles. She positions his head on a pillow, wraps a thick blanket around him, and places a towel under his cheek to catch his secretions.

"Relax," she says.

His eyes grow wide with fear.

"We won't go anywhere until you get used to it."

The next day, she tries again to secure him on the mattress. "You look comfortable."

He closes his eyes.

"Do you want to try going to the end of the driveway?"

He blinks twice. Yes.

She pushes the bed the short distance. "How was that? Should we go further?"

He blinks again. She walks the full length of the block, then around the corner.

"That went well," she tells Rick later that day.

The next afternoon, with John on the mobile bed ready for a long walk, she sees one of their dogs in the yard. "Should we take Rojo with us?"

He blinks fast.

Marianne ties the leash to the cart, then pushes it into the street like she did the day before. Blinded by the bright sun, she shields her eyes at the precise moment a cat jumps from a tree branch. Rojo rushes the cat, pulling the cart with him which sends John into the air with the mattress. He seems to fly in slow motion until he lands with the sound of an egg hitting the ground. She's afraid to look. As her hands blindly search his head for cuts or bruises, his shoulder bounces.

"Are you laughing?" She can't believe he thinks this is funny. "Let's go home."

At the house, Rojo wags his tail from the front porch. She rests John's hand on the dog's head.

"Next time, how about we leave him home?"

Later that night, she tells Rick what happened.

"Kids fall all the time," he says. "It's part of life."

She's startled by the truth of his words. Boys do get hurt. Her daughters also got hurt at the same age. When kids take risks, they're bound to get bruised. John is no different.

One weekend, they all play a game called "pie in the face." After each of them takes a turn, Marianne sprays whip cream in a pie tin and pushes it into John's face. She worries about clogging his nose prongs, but his left shoulder moves in laughter. He is happy, free and unrestrained by disease.

"More," he says.

Rick fills another pie plate with whipped cream. "Give our son what he wants."

"More," John says. Marianne laughs so hard she's ready to pass out.

Later she asks John a question that's become part of their bedtime routine. "Did you have a good day or a great day?" He answers the way he does each time she asks. "Me, too," she says. "I had a great day, too."

John uses flashcards to learn how to read. Math is not his thing; he's more of a Renaissance man who loves language and making art. He has a ranking system of stories he likes: mysteries followed by comedies, then science. He also likes realistic fiction. When he does artwork, I ask yes or no questions such as, do you want this color? He is very clear with yes or no. It's the first thing I told his mother: we have to get a clear yes/no. (Miss Laurie, teacher)

Are you kidding? This is the best job I have ever had. Three days a week, I drive ninety minutes from my house to get here and another hour and a half to get home. I'd do it every day if the school would allow it. John teases me because I'm the youngest of the J-Team. He makes me laugh all the time. I forget all my problems when I'm here. (Stephanie, speech therapist)

SEVEN YEARS OLD

A ROCK STAR LIKE SPRINGSTEEN

Amber and Britney, teenagers now, head off to the Jersey Shore the way she did at their age. Marianne understands their yearning. When life was dark and she was desperate for relief, the Jersey Shore saved her. The waves baptized her, leaving her cleansed. The sun bronzed her body, releasing impurities, and streaked her dark hair blond. At first, her mother permitted day trips but soon enough, she allowed Marianne to stay a full weekend with girlfriends, all of them sharing a cheap hotel room on the beach. The sun was never too hot, the waves never too big. Now, her favorite place in the world is her daughters' too.

"Go follow them," she tells Rick after the twins leave the

house one Friday night in a friend's car.

"You know they saw me last time I did this." He reaches for the keys. "I got all the way down to the Shore and when I stopped at a light, they crossed the street in front of the car. I slid way down in the seat but I'm sure they saw me."

Marianne laughs. "Please. Make sure they're safe."

"They're safe," Rick says. "It's New Jersey."

Again, she laughs. In his story, he saved her life by moving her to the New Jersey suburbs after they married. She swears he dragged her out of New York against her will. The truth is that she's more a Jersey girl than an Uptown girl, more Bruce Springsteen than Billy Joel. For her, flip-flops fit better than heels and shorts look better than skirts.

"We should all go to the Shore," Rick says.

"Are you serious?"

"Why not?" he says. "It's only two hours away."

"Well, John is more stable. He's old enough to help manage his breathing like Dr. Bach predicted. Unfortunately, he also knows how to stop himself from taking a breath and thinks it's funny."

She remembers the one night he stopped himself from taking a Bi-Pap breath. Where another in-rush of air should have been, there was none. The silence alerted her. She grabbed the Ambu-Bag and struggled with the mask. Her heart felt like it might rupture from fright then, all of a sudden, she saw his shoulder jump with laughter. When she was no longer bursting with anger at his prank, she explained to him why he must never do it again.

"Promise?" she said.

He closed his eyes, which she knew was no promise at all.

Before their weekend at the Shore, Marianne fills two suitcases with John's medical supplies, liquid nutrition, bathing suit and clothes. She makes room for the Bi-Pap and the suction machine. He will need everything on the road that he uses at home; she can't leave anything behind.

The twins bring a suitcase and Robby wears a backpack. Rick packs enough food for a week. Marianne grabs a bathing suit for herself on the way out. They leave early Friday afternoon to avoid traffic. Two hours later, the air is thick and heavy; she can smell the ocean from inside the car. They unpack, then drive to the boardwalk. The sun promises a few more hours of daylight. John lays on his mobile bed, strapped on for safety, his head elevated so he can look around. The computer sits in his lap. People pass from both directions.

"Hi," the computer says. "I'm John." He has the volume

turned way up. "What's your name?" He talks to every kid who walks by. Marianne rolls her eyes with embarrassment, but she knows he's hungry for friends his own age.

The twins throw balls at bowling pins for a top prize. Robby knocks down milk bottles. Rick aims a water pistol at a plastic clown. Standing a few feet away, a young boy stares at John. The first few times Marianne noticed people staring, she wanted to shoo them away. After a while, she realized they were curious, the way she was when she saw the boy in the wheelchair.

"Look Mommy," the boy says. "That kid brought his bed." The woman pulls the boy away.

"I'm so sorry."

"Don't worry about it," Marianne says. "John loves all the attention he can get." Later, she wonders if it's true.

"John, did you see that boy staring at you?"

"Ah huh."

"Does it bother you that he did that?"

He rolls his eyes.

"That's good," she says. "Do you know who else people stare at? Bruuuuuuuuuuuce." She stretches his name into a five-second syllable. Of course, John knows that name. Marianne blasts his music in the iPod she plays during their neighborhood walks. It's one of his favorite singers.

"Do you know why people stare at Bruce Springsteen?"

He rolls his eyes.

"Because Bruce is a rock star. That's why people stare at you John. Because you're a rock star like Bruce Springsteen." The way John pushes himself to do more and be more; that makes him a rock star. In one way, he's a bigger rock star than the Boss: John's eyes can make a computer talk; no way Bruce does that. She laughs at her silliness. Yet, she worries if she's doing the right thing by comparing John. Will he have an oversized ego because he thinks he's the Boss or will he simply see it as another measure of her love for him?

Early the next morning, she carries John towards the ocean. Along the way, she sheds the beach towel on the sand. She carries the Bi-Pap on one shoulder and an inflatable tube on the other. She holds John in her arms to the water's edge. There, he sits in the safety netting of the tube. Her idea is to walk him out a few feet, then let a soft wave carry him back to shore. Within seconds, however, a rogue wave capsizes him. She holds the Bi-Pap high above the water and pulls him out.

"That scared you, huh?" She lifts him into her arms, carries him up to the beach, and dries him off. "Please don't cry.

You'll get secretions and I don't have the machine with me." She carries him to the car. "You're going to be fine." She suctions him and changes him into dry clothes. "Sometimes a plan works out and other times, like now, it turns out to be a bad idea. You never know until you try." His eyes are wide and terrified. "Next time, I promise I'll be more prepared."

He rolls his eyes.

"What do you mean no next time? We'll try the bayside instead. There are no waves there."

In the morning, she gets him ready to go out in the water.

John rolls his eyes.

"Listen, John. You can't give up after one bad experience. If you don't keep trying, you'll never get where you want to go."

At the bay, she puts John in the same tube as yesterday. "Nothing to worry about." She holds on to the rope that's tied to the end of the tube. "I got you this time."

The rope grows taut as John floats away. She imagines this is how it will always be. John will venture out as far as he can, and she will help him get there. After a few minutes she pulls him in.

"Did you love it?"

His left shoulder bounces.

"Do you want more?"

"Ah huh."

Marianne chuckles. "Everyone should be so lucky."

On their last night, Rick takes them around the bay in a speedboat. She sits against the wheelhouse with John in her lap, both of them covered in wool blankets. Rick maneuvers the boat between the buoys, barely moving the water. Once the boat passes the markers furthest from the dock, he pushes the throttle.

"Faster," Marianne hollers into the wind. "Faster." The boat leaves twirls of water in its wake as the setting sun paints the sky red, orange and pink.

There's a photograph of our family at the Jersey Shore -- John, the twins, Robby, me, Marianne -- and we're all smiling. Everyone's happy. I can sum up that scene in one sentence. You do your best in a difficult situation and life goes on. (Rick)

SEVEN TO NINE YEARS OLD

BEGIN AGAIN

"Don't cry, John. I don't have time to suction you." His face is wet with tears. "Please stop." She wipes his cheeks. "Uncle Robert's daughter is getting married. I have to go."

The night nurse rushes in. "Sorry I'm late." She wipes her nose with a crumpled tissue. "Traffic."

"Do you have a cold?" Marianne says.

"Allergies."

"Are you sure? I can stay, you know."

The nurse sneezes into her hand. "I forgot to take my medication. I'm fine."

Rick honks the horn.

"John, Mommy is leaving." She kisses his head. "You can watch videos until we get back."

In the car, a bad feeling haunts her. During the reception, her stomach rages. Later, when they return home, John is sick. He struggles to breathe because his airways are clogged with phlegm and secretions. His oxygen count is low. His eyes are red.

I should never have left him.

Marianne pushes the red tube into his mouth, down his throat, and into his upper airways. The suction machine gurgles as it vacuums up secretions. The cough assist pulls from the lower airways, bringing up more gunk. Then, one last sweep with the red tube. She repeats this respiratory treatment every two hours throughout the night.

In the morning, he isn't any better so the pediatrician sends a nurse with antibiotics. Later in the day, Robert brings Vera home after a few days at his house.

"What's wrong?" Vera says.

"We have to keep a close eye on John. He's got a cold." John's condition worsens over the next few hours.

"He doesn't look good," Rick says.

"You're right. We can't wait any longer."

"Robert," Marianne yells. "Call 9-1-1."

A few minutes later, he stands at the doorway to John's room with a jacket in his hand. "An ambulance is on the way." His brow is wrinkled with worry. "I'm going outside for some air."

She squeezes the Ambu-Bag to force air into John's lungs, but his airways are too blocked for the manual pressure. Marianne isn't sure what to do. *Please, Dad, help me.* Then she has a thought. Instead of using the Ambu-Bag, what if she changes the settings on the cough assist, to blow out air instead of suctioning. She tries that on John. When she sees his chest rise, she knows he has a chance. *Thank you, Dad.*

When the EMTs arrive, they take over. Marianne follows them into the ambulance. As they race to the hospital, she remembers the dream she had about her Dad. He visited her almost every night for years up until John was born. He was always dressed in a tuxedo, handsome and young. They laughed and played together. Whenever it was time for him to leave, she would grab hold of his jacket.

"Take me with you."

He kissed her head. "I can't. You have something big to do here." He knew John would need her long before she did.

"We're taking him local," the EMT says. "He's too sick for anything else." During the ride, John's eyes roll behind his lids.

"John, open your eyes." Marianne puts her face close to his. "Look at Mommy, John. If you close your eyes, you won't see Mommy anymore." His eyes open and find her face. "That's it, John. Look at Mommy."

In the emergency room, Rick arrives as the doctor diagnoses John. "He has double pneumonia. We have to intubate."

Marianne calls the girls at college. "John is very sick," she tells them. "The doctors are doing everything they can for your brother, but it's very bad."

When Robert visits the hospital, John's diagnosis devastates him. "It's the worst thing that could happen. There's no way he can make it this time." The next morning, he is shocked his nephew survived the night. "It defies everything I've ever been taught."

John's doctor remains cautious. "We still have to take care of the pneumonia."

"What about his respiratory treatments?" Marianne says. "He needs a special protocol followed twice a day."

"Our nurses will handle that, but curing the pneumonia is our first priority."

Lulled into a sense of security, they let the doctor take charge and resume the same routine as before: Marianne with John in the hospital; Rick at home with the other children and Vera.

"I can't believe we're doing this again," she says.

"John looks worse than I've ever seen him," Rick says.

Each day, nurses thump John's back like Vera did years ago, but they don't suction him or use a cough assist. One evening towards the end of John's first week in ICU, a nurse tiptoes into the room where Marianne and Rick sit with their son.

"Why are you here?" she says. "I'm nervous saying this, but I can't keep quiet any longer. I used to work with Dr. Bach. You really need to take your son to him." Marianne looks at Rick, dumbfounded they hadn't realized it sooner.

"He'll ask why we waited so long," Rick says.

"We'll tell him the truth. We thought John was in good hands. We were wrong."

At the Emergency Room in the Newark hospital John is admitted under Dr. Bach's care. Hours later, he takes them to John's bedside. "It took multiple tries, but he's on the Bi-Pap again with the nose prongs." John stares at them, his eyes soulful.

"You can hold him," Dr. Bach says.

She doesn't dare. Yet how can she not? Marianne lifts John into her arms. She rests her face on his cheek and closes her eyes, inhaling his essence. He is delicate, like a feather that blows in a breeze. "You are more beautiful than ever," she whispers. "I think maybe you are an angel."

His eyes find hers.

"I knew it. You are an angel, John. You are the brightest in the entire universe."

For five days, Marianne hovers over John like she did in the days after his diagnosis. Each time the oxygen level dips low, she thinks she could lose him and herself. Adrenaline floods her, but fear paralyzes her.

Dr. Bach reassures her. "Give him time. He will get stronger and stronger."

She knows her anxiety won't help John so she acts as if everything is okay. She talks to herself about faith even as she questions her own. She visualizes John at home, watching videos, floating in the therapy pool, and exercising with Rashida.

"Is John any better?" Rick asks her one morning.

"I'll settle for stable." She doesn't want to offer false hope.

"That's good enough for me," he says.

Dr. Bach's respiratory treatments help John, and he does get better. He gains back some of the weight he lost and his skin looks healthy. His eyes are again curious. After a few more days of recovery, Dr. Bach is ready to discharge him.

"Are you sure?" Marianne says.

"He will improve at home as much as here."

She doesn't understand his faith in her. She certainly doesn't trust herself.

There first day home, Marianne gets a telephone call from the hospital doctor. "I wanted to check on your son."

She's heard that tone before from doctors who presume John wouldn't make it. "John is here with me," she says.

"What?"

"He's doing well." She tries to keep her voice pleasant.

"How?" the doctor asks. "He was so sick."

"Dr. John Bach saved him."

"Who is this doctor? How do I reach him? I need to learn what he knows."

She wants to be angry at the man for assuming John was gone, but what's the point? John is home and there are things to be done. She gives the contact information to the doctor and hangs up.

The other children are happy John is home. They huddle in his room, rarely leaving his side. Marianne hates to be away from him; even food shopping is too long to be gone. It is not an easy time for her and Rick. They are not neglecting each other on purpose, but John needs so much, and there is so little left over for each other at the end of the day.

Rashida begins to work with John again. She comes to the house every day, carefully moving his legs and arms. Marianne puts him in the water, an hour a day, just like before. She is not sure he can handle that but Rashida encourages her. "If you don't try, you never know." From then on, Rashida is always around, doing some little exercise with John. She sings to him. "You are a trooper. You are strong. You are the best."

When John gets healthier and is ready for more, Rashida uses the passive stationary bike with pedals strapped to his feet. Later, Marianne attaches the pedals to John's hands and uses the machine to exercise his arms. He starts off slow, and only for a few minutes at the beginning.

The J-Team works together to move his body and invigorate his mind. Each day repeats itself with more exercises. John pushes himself, sweating and grunting. He accumulates milestones of time in the Stander. More treatments, including electromagnetic stimulation and vibrating machines, are added. After a few months, he sits up with the soft brace, yoga blocks and rolled towels. With each passing day, John grows stronger. Marianne grows stronger too, and she is less afraid. She refuses to succumb to negative thoughts and feels better when she is hopeful about John's life. It's not always easy but she knows it's the only way to live. All the other problems of the world fade away when she sees how hard he works to stay alive and get stronger.

It takes two years before John fully recovers from the double pneumonia. During that time, Marianne tries to maintain a happy family life for the children and Rick. The girls are back in college, and Robby is now in middle school. If asked, Marianne would say this has been a turning point for her. Seeing her brother open up and hearing the doctor so shocked at the miracle of John's life led to a shift in her thinking.

"Things will be different from now on," she tells Rick. "I'm not going to take another day with John for granted. Whatever happens, happens, but I am not going to worry all the time. Having John alive today is a miracle, and I'm going to enjoy it even if it's the last day with him."

After all we went through with John, I'm amazed Rick and I are together. The years after John's pneumonia were the worst; I had one way of seeing things and he had another. People told me they took bets on when we would split up. I had to do some heavy-duty soul searching if we had any hope of surviving as husband and wife. I knew I had to change and make space for his way of seeing things and doing things. Thankfully, we both agreed that whatever best served the family was good enough for each of us. With a shared vision, we moved to a place of mutual respect no matter what happened or what either of us said. There is power in that kind of love. (Marianne)

I don't discuss my personal feelings. Marianne likes to talk things out, but I'm not that way. (Rick)

TEN TO TWELVE YEARS OLD

LIVING LARGE

For a long time, Marianne hasn't wanted to take John out, but she can tell that he is bored and wants to do things. She remembers Dr. Bach cautioned them about being over-protective and also remembers her promise to enjoy each moment with him. Now it's time for him to have as much life experience as possible.

"I want him to have a taste of what the other kids are having," she says. Rick agrees. He doesn't want to hold John back any more than the disease requires.

After years of physical therapy, John is strong enough for the wheelchair that Marianne jury-rigs to fit his frame, giving him more freedom than he's ever had. Challenged by the new experience, John can only sit in the wheelchair for a few minutes at a time. She encourages him to push his endurance further.

"Imagine the places we can go with the wheelchair instead of the mobile bed. The baseball field to watch Robby play. The bookstore to pick out a best seller."

As he gains confidence in his ability, John is able to go places he's never been before. One Sunday, Rick takes the family to a restaurant where the chef prepares food at tableside. Another time she takes the boys to the Liberty Science Center and Planetarium, where John sits in her lap to ride a simulator that takes them on a train. He wants more.

After John manages a few events in his wheelchair, they all go to the Mall to see one of their favorite monsters, Godzilla, on the big screen. They take the indoor elevator up four floors to the theater. After the movie opens, the fire alarm blasts from the speakers and everyone is directed to leave the building.

"Go," Marianne tells the girls. "Take Robby with you. We'll meet you outside."

"No way," Britney says.

"We leave together," Amber says.

"Definitely," says Robby.

She turns to Rick.

"Don't look at me. I'm not leaving either."

Several men gather around John. "The elevator isn't working. We can help carry the wheelchair down the stairs," one says. People make room for them to pass as they carry John to the Mall exit. Marianne stops to let a few people out first.

"You go," a woman says. "We'll leave after your family."

"Thank you so much," Marianne says.

Outside, she stands with John among the crowd.

"Angels are all around us, John. All we have to do is open our eyes."

When the Make-A-Wish Foundation asks John to pick the place he would most love to visit, he chooses the Kaufman Astoria Studios in Queens, New York, television home to Sesame Street. Fascinated by Jim Henson's Muppets from an early age, he studies how they move and express emotion. He loves the technical aspects of puppeteering and the history of the show, but there's nothing like seeing them in action. Marianne and the twins can't wait to go with him.

At the Studio, John's name shines in lights on a sign above the door. Inside, puppets rush towards them. John shakes with excitement. The computer sits in his lap. One man pulls a chair next to John. He is tall with curly hair that falls past his shoulders. His puppet is the wonderful, larger-than-life wooly mammoth named Snuffleupagus.

"Hi. I'm Marty Robinson."

"John knows who you are. We all do." Marianne shakes the man's hand. Bert and Ernie say hello, then Kermit the frog, John's favorite. Marianne thinks this might be the best day of his life so far. The crew invites John to watch them shoot a scene, then begs him to stay for lunch. With his initial shyness gone, John asks all the questions he loaded into the computer at home.

When their scheduled time is up, no one wants them to leave. The puppet, Abby Cadabby, sits close to John. Abby waves her magic wand around his head.

"We've been sucked into the world of John's love," her puppeteer, Leslie Carrara-Rudolph, says.

The first rumors about SMA treatments and gene therapy surfaced when John was seven or eight. Since then, something new always seemed to be in the works, but nothing materialized. Plenty of times, Marianne worried about the delay. *What if there is no miracle drug? What if no treatment is developed? What are we doing to this kid?* That's when she gave herself a reality check. *Look at all this boy does and all the people who love him. He has a full life.*

Now, there's hot news about a clinical trial scheduled in Boston for a new drug called Nusinersen, also known as Spinraza. From what she's heard, Spinraza targets a back-up gene and increases production of a protein needed for the muscles to work.

She packs them both a suitcase.

"We're going to Boston, John. A cure is coming and it could happen any day now."

He speaks a series of sounds.

"You want to know how we should tell Grandma that you have been cured?"

"Ah huh."

"What do you think we should do?"

He utters more sounds.

Marianne laughs. "You want to surprise her?"

He blinks twice.

"Oh, she'll love that."

While they wait for more information, John continues to train. Each day, he starts with Dr. Bach's respiratory treatment. Then, he attends school and completes his occupational therapy. After that, he's in the water with Marianne. In the evening, Rashida works out with him and after that, the stationary bike exercises his legs and the rower exercises each of his arms. In between it all, he spends time in the Stander, his least favorite exercise.

"Would you like to practice walking?" Marianne asks him one day.

"Ah huh."

John sits in Marianne's lap while Rashida wraps extra-wide bandages around them both, from underneath his armpits to his waist. She helps Marianne stand with John attached, and wraps more bandages around their bellies, hips, and thighs. His feet don't sit directly on top of hers, so Rashida ties their ankles together instead.

Marianne holds his head with one hand and balances with the other like a gymnast on a balance beam. He's nearly eighty-seven pounds and five-foot-three, so it will be a work-out for both of them. She digs deep for a breath and takes a step forward. John's body tenses as his leg muscles feel every ounce of his weight. They walk together to the kitchen and back. It feels like they have run an entire marathon.

"You are a champion," Marianne tells him. "A real hero."

During the clinical trial, children with SMA who are given Spinraza reach important milestones. They are able to turn over on their own. They can sit up without help. They also show improvement in breathing, and in neck and back control. The drug is so effective that the clinical trial is stopped and all participants receive the treatment.

When Rick hears the news, he contacts a doctor he met early in his SMA research who's now involved in the drug's development. "Is this really happening?"

"It's what we've all been waiting for," the doctor says.

"I want my son to get this drug. What do we need to do for that to happen?"

"Be patient. It won't be much longer."

Spinraza is fast-tracked through the U.S. Food and Drug Administration and approved as the first treatment for SMA in December 2016. John's pediatrician is beyond ecstatic when he hears the news.

"You did it," he tells Marianne.

"No," she says. "We all did it."

The same way I tell Amber, Britney, and Robby, I tell John: if you want something bad enough, you have to keep working at it. 'Never give up,' I tell them. 'Never give up,' I tell myself. It's the only way to live. (Marianne)

THIRTEEN TO FOURTEEN YEARS OLD

OLYMPIC MOMENTS

The New York City hospital where baby John spent three months will soon offer Spinraza treatments in its SMA clinic. Marianne calls them days after the FDA approves the drug.

"When can my son get his first dose?"

"Someone will be in contact with you soon," the receptionist tells her.

When no one calls after a week, Marianne wraps John in blankets and secures his wheelchair in the van. She looks at him through the rearview mirror.

"We can't just sit around and wait, right?"

"Ah huh."

In the clinic, she stands impatiently at the front desk, waiting for the receptionist to finish a phone call.

"I want to make an appointment for my son to receive his first Spinraza treatment."

The receptionist looks up John's information

"There are 250 babies on the waiting list. The most fragile go first. Your son won't be seen for months."

The irony is not lost on Marianne. John pushed himself all these years to stay healthy and strong for a cure. Now that it's here, he's too strong for the front of the line.

"I'm sorry," the nurse says. "He'll just have to wait."

"He's waited a very long time and shouldn't have to wait any longer. None of the children should have to wait. They've been through enough."

Marianne and John head toward the elevator when another nurse rushes up to them.

"I hear there's no waiting list at the SMA clinic in Morristown, New Jersey. You should call them." When she telephones the clinic, John is able to get an appointment.

"All they need is the insurance company's approval," she tells Rick that night.

"I'm not sure we'll get it," he says. "Spinraza is seven

hundred fifty thousand dollars for the first year. Maintenance doses are a hundred twenty-five thousand dollars each. Those are big numbers."

"It sounds astronomical but think about it," Marianne says. "People spent more than ten years researching and testing. They absolutely deserve to be paid."

Rick isn't surprised when John's claim for treatment is denied. "Every time we tried for something new, they said no. We need to appeal." John's pediatrician writes an official letter of need, while Marianne pens her own plea.

My son was born with the inherited neuromuscular disease called Spinal Muscular Atrophy (SMA). John has the most severe type (type1). Babies born with SMA type 1 develop symptoms before birth or in the first few months of life and usually die before their second birthday. John cannot eat, breathe, swallow, or move on his own. Until recently, our only wishes for John were for him to feel as loved as humanly possible, keep him relatively pain-free and have his whole family by his side when the time came that his flaccid body could take no more. Because of this drug, my son has a chance to live a life all parents imagine for their children. Please, I implore you as a mother, approve this drug for my son so that he can have a future and a life he so longs for.

When she can wait no longer, Marianne telephones the insurance company. "I need to speak with someone about the claim for Spinraza for our son."

"I'm sorry, ma'am, the claim was rejected."

"I know but we appealed." Her pulse quickens.

"I'm sorry but the claim was rejected again."

She grips the phone. "I want to speak to the person who made the decision. Otherwise, I will bundle up my child in his wheelchair, with his feeding tube and breathing machine, and come to your office. Then I'll find this person so he or she can look John in the eyes and tell him to his face why he does not deserve this life-saving treatment." She touches the throbbing vein in her neck. Any semblance of calm is gone.

"Hold on," the woman says.

Marianne tries to steady her breathing.

"Hello?" the woman says. "Are you there?"

"Yes, I'm here," Marianne says.

"The procedure is approved for your son."

"Seriously?" She says a prayer of thanksgiving.

"Yes. A letter will go out today."

John rolls his eyes when she tells him the news.

"You don't want to get the shot? Why not?"

He answers with familiar sounds and tones.

"You're afraid of the hospital?"

He blinks twice.

"Because you remember the bad things that happened?"

"Ah huh."

"This time will be different. We'll have a sleepover. Grandma will be there. Your sisters will be there. We'll have fun."

In the hospital on the day of John's first Spinraza treatment, Marianne suctions his airways. With the nurse's help, they flip John onto his belly. Marianne supports his head so he can watch the video monitor next to his bed. She can tell he's as nervous as she is.

"You'll be able to see everything that's happening," she says, unsure if that's good or not. "Don't worry. I'm here." She tries to ignore her own building anxiety.

The radiologist locates the precise place on John's spine to inject the drug. He numbs the area and inserts a medical port for the injection. A doctor then administers the drug by withdrawing five milliliters of spinal fluid and then replacing it with five milliliters of Spinraza. When the procedure is completed, the port is removed.

"Your son must lay on his back without moving for one

hour so we can monitor him."

"No problem. John's not much of a mover."

Amber and Britney decorate John's hospital room with a Snuffleupagus puppet from the gift shop and bright signs to congratulate him.

That night, John's oxygen numbers hold steady between ninety-eight and one hundred.

"That's a good sign," the doctor says. Yet, she urges patience. "He is older and taller than the children in the clinical trial, so the drug has to travel further. It's all unchartered territory."

"You don't know John. He's been working toward this moment his entire life."

AUGUST 8, 2002

When you think you're going to lose your child, there's nothing worse in the world. When Spinraza came out, it was a rebirth, a miracle. In my heart of hearts, I knew Spinraza would help John. He was ready. (Marianne)

FIFTEEN YEARS OLD

THE KIDS ARE ALRIGHT

"Can you believe it? Two whole months at the Shore."

"I'll believe it when we're there," Rick says. "We came close last summer, too."

"John is more stable this year."

"When is school over?"

"Today's the last day. Tonight, he has play rehearsal."

Rick laughs. "I remember his last play at the school."

"Shrek, right? He played Daddy Dwarf. Or was that when he was the football player?" Marianne laughs. "He was so funny in both shows."

"Anything else on his to-do list?"

"One more shot this week and that's it."

"Like I said, I'll believe it when we're on the beach."

"We have to go. It's our last summer with Robby. After senior year, he won't want family vacations."

"Do you think the girls will come?"

"Are you kidding? They already made plans with their girlfriends to come with us."

That afternoon, the J-Team sticks around longer than usual after they finish their work with John.

"Make sure your mother reads to you," Miss Laurie says.

Marianne rolls her eyes. "It's summer vacation."

"I'll visit as often as I can," Joan says.

"That's wonderful. Come any time you want."

John interrupts with a series of sounds.

"No, you can't watch videos right now. First, you have one more session with Rashida."

John focuses his eyes on the computer screen.

"I feel sick," the computer says. "My stomach hurts. I need to rest."

"That's too funny." Marianne looks around at the J-Team. "Who helped him program those phrases?" Giggling, the women look away. "Oh, I see how it is." When she looks to John for the answer, he closes his eyes. "You are all thick as thieves."

Stephanie makes a list of tasks for his summer break. "The biggest thing, John, is the computer. Use it and talk to people."

"Please, don't encourage him. He carries it on the boardwalk and talks to everyone."

John lasers his eyes on a different block of words until they are highlighted. "I want attention. I want attention."

At the Shore, Marianne shifts to a slower pace. The warm air revitalizes her and the hot sun lightens her load. She starts John's day with his respiratory treatment -- nebulizer, cough assist, suction, and ends his day the same way. John exercises with the stationary bike, the rower, and the Stander, and he works out with Rashida three times a week. Each day, he spends ninety minutes in the pool. Daily water therapy is as critical to John's health as his respiratory treatments. Otherwise, his muscles contract and his body tightens. The rest of the time, John is on vacation, too. At night, he hangs out with Robby watching YouTube while his brother plays video games until Marianne yells at them to stop.

"It's three a.m. Go to bed." She tries to sound angry but loves that her boys are as normal as other teenagers who stay up all night and sleep till noon.

One night when Robby is out with friends, Marianne sits

in John's room. "What do you want to watch?" She scrolls through the video app on his tablet until he stops her. "Okay, here you go." She settles into the chair to watch a television show they began days ago.

A minute later, he makes a familiar sound.

"You want a repeat?"

"Ah huh." When the show ends, he asks to see it again.

"Are you kidding John? When do I get a turn to watch one of my shows?" She sets the kitchen timer for five minutes. "This is the absolute last repeat."

He lets out a long series of sounds.

"No, I won't call Robby. Yes, I know he would let you repeat and repeat. Fine, one more time."

When John turns fifteen that August, they throw him a birthday party at the Shore. Rick buys food and invites his parents. Robert brings Vera. Marianne bakes a cake and slides a DVD through the middle. She started this gag years ago and continues every birthday, though he's no longer surprised or amused. She wraps gifts -– a Monster Truck and a behind-the-scenes table book about Sesame Street. The twins hang a piñata. Robby hands out confetti poppers. They sing Happy Birthday as John is wheeled into the living room, and pop confetti. His shoulder bounces as colorful paper rains on him.

Britney stands behind her brother. "Do you want to hit the pinata John?" She helps him hold the stick.

"Wait," Marianne says. "Blindfold him first."

With his eyes covered and Britney helping him hold the stick, John misses the piñata over and over.

"Here, let me try," Britney says. With one hit, she breaks open the piñata. Candy and trinkets scatter across the floor.

The next morning, Marianne shuffles into the kitchen for coffee. Soon, the twins join her, fixing their own morning brew. As she watches her daughters, one part of her sees that they are beautiful young women who live full lives; another part wonders if she raised them okay.

"How was your childhood?"

"Where did that come from?" Amber asks. "We haven't even had coffee yet."

"We're fine," Britney says. "There are no lingering resentments or bad feelings."

"We have always felt loved," Amber says. "Honestly."

Robby walks in, rubbing his eyes. Marianne jumps up and reaches for his arm. "Let's do the Robby dance. The Robby dance. Let's do the Robby dance."

Robby groans. "You can stop now."

"How was your childhood?"

"The best of all my friends. No one had as much fun."

Marianne kisses him.

"I love you too, Mom. Can you fix me some food?"

After breakfast, the twins' mood turn serious. "There's something we want to talk to you about," Amber says. "If something happens to you and Rick, Britney and I want to be the ones to take care of John."

Marianne wasn't expecting this.

"Nothing's going to happen," she says. "I exercise and eat right, so I'm going to live a long time. Rick's younger than me, so no worries there either."

"This is important, Mom," Britney says.

"No one else needs to worry about John. He's my responsibility to take care of."

"He's our brother," Amber says. "He's supposed to be with us, and we would want to take care of him."

"I'm in on that," Robby says.

Now I have to face all three.

"Listen, I appreciate what you're saying, but you will want

to marry and start your own families."

"John is our family," Britney says.

Marianne tries another tactic. "John doesn't want to live with anyone but me."

"You might be surprised," Amber says.

Later that day, she tells Rick about the conversation. "Caring for John is 24/7," she says. "I can't put all of that responsibility on the kids."

"I know it's hard, but if that's what they want."

"You agree with them?"

"They're siblings. Don't they belong together?"

"What about John? What about what he wants?"

"Have you asked him?"

"I'll ask when he's older."

"He's fifteen. How much older does he need to be?"

Marianne remembers when Dr. Bach said John might want to live on his own one day. That night, she asks John about it.

"Do you think you will get married someday?"

"Ah huh."

"If you get married, will you let Mommy live with you and your wife?"

He blinks twice.

"If your wife says no, will you stay married to her?"

He rolls his eyes.

She may as well ask what she most wants to know. "Do you have a secret plan to live with your brother and sisters?"

He closes his eyes.

She should have seen it coming. After he received his last maintenance dose of Spinraza, he asked her to leave while he lay unmoving for an hour of monitoring. When she returned after several minutes, he spoke the word she is most familiar with.

"More."

"You want me to leave again?"

"Ah huh." His loudest shout for independence until now.

One afternoon John asks Marianne to take him for a walk around the neighborhood.

"It's raining, John. Let's wait till it stops."

He whines and asks again.

"No, I can't go right now."

He sounds out a sentence.

"Fine, the nurse can take you." She looks to the day nurse. "Do you mind a walk in the rain?"

When they return, John's eyes are red with tears.

"He cried the whole way because you didn't go with him,"

the nurse says.

Marianne slips the red tube between his lips and down his throat. The suction machine gurgles as it clears his upper airways. She uses the cough assist to reach his lower airways.

"Are you okay now, John?" she asks.

"Ah huh."

"Are you sure?"

He blinks twice.

"Now you listen here. You are old enough to know what happens if you cry when you're away from the machines." She doesn't like to yell, but sometimes it's the only way to get through to her children. John is no different. When Rick gets home, she tells him what happened. He pulls up a chair next to John and leans in.

"Did you get in trouble, Johnny?" Rick is the only one he lets call him that.

"Ah huh."

"You want me to talk to Mom for you?"

"Ah huh."

Marianne is struck by the tenderness between them. "You always take his side," she teases.

"Because he's a lot like me."

"You can't take credit for all his qualities."

"He's stubborn. That one's on you."

Since John's Sprinraza treatments, Marianne looks for nuances of change in his body. She also looks to see that he is happy. He laughs at everything, and has a list of things people can do to entertain him: act like a dying person, pretend you are choking on something, fall into the Christmas tree.

Like any teenager, he wants more movies and better technology. And he wants more friends. He wants play dates. He wants a social life with kids his own age.

"Try not to be nervous, John." Marianne smooths his hair. "You rehearsed a lot with Aunt Kathie." Rick's youngest sister walks over.

"You know what to do," Kathie says. "You've got this. Don't worry." The dancers gather on stage as the audience settles down. The idea started as a game of imagination.

"Let's make up a dance," Kathie told John a few years ago. "You'll be the audience and I'll dance for you." They pretended like this until one day they decided to have an actual dance recital. The first year John was in the audience. The second year, he delivered opening remarks. This year, he will make a speech.

As the spotlight frames John, the computer speaks the words he wrote with the J-Team's help.

"Hi everyone. Thank you for coming out today. I want to start off with a joke. Why is 8 afraid of 7? He waits a beat. "Because 7, 8, 9."

The audience laughs. Marianne laughs, too, though she's heard the joke dozens of times. Seven ate nine. She laughs harder. *You're as funny as your Uncle Robert. A real entertainer.*

"It's nothing short of a miracle that I feel so many changes happening in my body."

Amen to that. He's prepared all his life for this miracle. Every day, ninety minutes in the therapy pool, forty-five minutes on bike, an hour in the Stander, an hour of whole-body vibrations. Physical therapy, occupational therapy, speech therapy. Every. Single. Day.

Sometimes she looks back and wonders how she is still breathing. It wasn't easy, but she wouldn't want it any other way. Their lifestyle is full of drama and not all of it is good. It's not for everyone but it works for her family. John is the glue that keeps them together. Comfortable in his skin, he is cut from different cloth than her. He knows what he wants while she frequently second guesses herself.

The audience is quiet as John's computer continues to speak his words. "I know it will take a lot more time, hard work and support before I can do many of the things I dream about, but I am ready for the challenge. To go where no man has gone before."

"Boldly," she whispers. "You go boldly where no man has gone before." Marianne tries not to cry as the audience gives him a standing ovation.

John's left shoulder bounces with excitement.

THE KIDS ARE ALRIGHT

When I look back, I feel that there was a bigger plan than I could imagine and a Higher Power leading the way. (Marianne)

SEVENTEEN YEARS OLD

REAL-LIFE WONDER BOY

John Del Guercio, in his own words:

What's the hardest thing about having SMA1?

"To see everyone else walking and moving and eating and even though I try hard, I can't."

What makes you happiest?

"Watching YouTube makes me happiest because I can become the character I am watching and pretend I am doing what everyone else is."

How would you describe yourself?

"I am a boy who has weak muscles and wears a Bi-Pap, but is like everyone else."

What's your favorite color?

"Red."

What do you love most of all?

"My mom because she is the best mom in the world."

What's your advice to parents of a child with SMA1?

"Be kind and patient and have fun."

What are your favorite things to do?

"I love doing anything fun with my family and watching Sesame Street."

How do you feel about a book about your life?

"I love it. It's important that people know what it's like to live with this disease."

I asked John all of the questions, and his answers made me really tear up. (Marianne)

Acknowledgements

ACKNOWLEDGEMENTS

MARIANNE DEL GUERCIO

I would like to express my gratitude for the many miracles bestowed upon me. God, Allah, Jehovah, the Universe: thank you for seeing in me, what for my whole life, I couldn't. Thank you to my husband, Rick. Thank you to the four miracles we call our children; you are my greatest gifts and my true reason for living. Thanks to my mother, who stayed by my side and taught me to react no matter how frightening a situation, and to my father, for coming through from the other side and holding my hand when I needed him most. Thanks to my brothers, sisters-in-law, brothers-in-law, nieces, nephews, cousins, friends, and neighbors, for your support over the years. To John's teacher, therapists, and devoted nurses, thank you for seeing ability, not disability; all of you are my village. Make no mistake, we accomplished this together. I also thank the doctors who encouraged us and went way beyond the call of duty: Dr. John Bach, Dr. Jahannaz Dastgir, and Dr. William Middlesworth; without you, there would no longer be a John or a Marianne.

To Judith Conte, my cousin, my friend and my storyteller, thank you for spending countless days, weeks, months and beyond with me and my unique family. You left your home and your own family, traveled across the country and lived meagerly with mine, trying hard not to "intrude" so you could get every detail and tell an accurate story of a boy who beat the odds. You, too, are a hero in this story.

And finally, to John. I am so grateful you picked me to be your Mommy and taught me what a hero truly looks like. I can't wait until we cross the finish line of your first half-marathon. I love you from the earth to the moon, to the stars, to the planets, to Heaven, and back home again!

ACKNOWLEDGEMENTS

JUDITH A. CONTE

Thank you, John Del Guercio, for inviting me into your life and becoming my friend. You are living proof.

Thank you, my cousin, Marianne, for saying yes to an idea and remaining faithful to the result. Thank you, Rick, for welcoming me into your home for weeks at a time. Thank you Amber, Britney and Robby for letting me eavesdrop on your lives. You all made this book possible. Special thanks to Vera Brescia, my aunt and earliest role model of beauty, courage and love.

Thanks Robert, for sharing insight; to Laurie for details about your research; and to Kathie for anecdotes about ballet recitals with John. Thank you, Dr. Bach, for teaching me your protocol. Thank you Karen, Patti, Jeannie, and Manny, for adding texture to the story. Thanks to the J-Team for letting me watch. Thanks to my sisters for sharing memories.

Thank you, *all meh chil'ren dem*, for believing in me. Chloe Mae, thanks for the gorgeous author photo and your early imaginings of what this book could look like. William Carlos, my favorite son, thank you for reading early versions and encouraging me to finish. Tahnee Jo, my wildly talented youngest, thank you for the brilliant suggestion on chapter structure; your idea made this a much better book.

A big shout out to Alaska friends: Lila, for editing with sharp eyes and a generous heart; Joanie and Brenda, for keeping me on the straight and narrow; Vered for good coffee and thoughtful publishing advice.

Humble and earnest thanks to the amazing people who bought advance copies of the book and waited patiently for its delivery. Knowing you were there, waiting for your copy, pushed me when I most needed it. Thanks, also, to everyone who scooped up beta copies and offered opinions.

Most heart-felt thanks to Teresa Donati, Ulla Neuburger, and Silvino da Silva, my life-long friends. Terri, your brilliance shines a bright light on my world, reminding me of all the good that surrounds me. Ulla, thank you for sharing your home and island life with me; it's been the adventure of my lifetime. Silvino, thank you for carrying this project over the finish line; with you at the helm of Mighty Acorn Press, this book became real.

ABOUT THE AUTHOR

JUDITH A. CONTE

Judith lives in Anchorage, Chicago, and St. Croix where she shares life with family and friends. While she worked as a lawyer in a day job, Judith wrote a memoir about her life in the U.S. Virgin Islands in the 1980's titled, *Paradise Blown*, and a screenplay of the same name. During her time in St. Croix, Judith was also senior writer for the travel and tourism publication *The Croixer*. In Alaska she wrote a divorce advice column, a series of newspaper vignettes on community life in Anchorage, and helped create *Anchorage Remembers: An Anthology of Alaskan Writers Celebrating the Centennial, 1915-2015.*

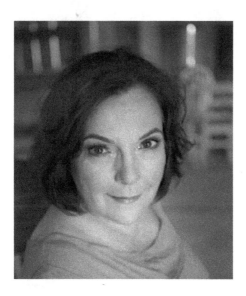

CPSIA information can be obtained
at www.ICGtesting.com
Printed in the USA
LVHW040058180122
708503LV00005B/444